BUMPALICIOUS

BUMPALICIOUS

How to relax and enjoy your pregnancy

by Denise Van Outen

Nutrition consultant: Amanda Ursell
Fitness consultant: Nicki Waterman
Edited by Sam Mann

headline

Nutrition consultant: Amanda Ursell
Fitness consultant: Nicki Waterman
Edited by Sam Mann

First published in 2011
by HEADLINE PUBLISHING GROUP

1

Cataloguing in Publication Data is available from the British Library

ISBN 978 0 7553 6172 4

Typeset in Formata and Sabon by Perfect Bound Ltd

Illustrations by Montana Forbes

Printed in the UK by Butler Tanner and Dennis Ltd

Headline's policy is to use papers that are natural, renewable and
recyclable products and made from wood grown in sustainable forests.
The logging and manufacturing processes are expected to conform to the
environmental regulations of the country of origin.

HEADLINE PUBLISHING GROUP
An Hachette UK Company
338 Euston Road
London NW1 3BH

www.headline.co.uk
www.hachette.co.uk

Contents

Editors' Introduction

Every pregnancy is different – and yours is no exception. This book is a record of Denise's own personal journey, so don't worry if your pregnancy does not correspond exactly to hers. Unfortunately, space does not allow every subject to be covered in this volume – so if you are carrying twins or multiple babies, or have specific health concerns, then you should always consult your medical practitioner before taking any of the general advice in this book.

Each chapter in *Bumpalicious* is divided into three parts: an overview of what is going on in your body that month, Denise's diary recording her experiences, and expert nutritional and fitness advice from Amanda Ursell and Nicki Waterman. Not every subject corresponds to a specific month – swollen ankles, for example, can strike at any time – so do use the index at the back if you want to look up a particular subject.

Finally, you'll notice that your baby is referred to as 'he' in the general sections – this is just to avoid the use of 'he/she', though obviously all the advice refers to those carrying girls as well as boy babies!

Meet the Team

Denise Van Outen needs no introduction…

Amanda Ursell studied nutrition at King's College, London University and has a degree in nutrition and a post-graduate diploma in dietetics. She is an award-winning writer, author and television presenter and has weekly columns in *The Times*, the *Sun* and *Buzz Magazine* and a monthly column and contributions in *Healthy* magazine and *Spirit & Destiny*, making her the most widely read nutritionist in the UK. Previous long-running columns include *The Sunday Times Style Magazine*, *The Los Angeles Times* and *Harpers Baazar*. She has been the nutrition editor on *Sainsbury's* and *Men's Health* magazines and edited *Well Being* magazine for two years. A regular presenter on the *Tonight* programme, Amanda was *GMTV's* resident nutritionist for twelve years.

Nicki Waterman is one of the country's most high-profile and highly respected fitness experts. She regularly appears on television and in the national press, including her weekly 'Fit Squad' column for the *Sun* and monthly columns for *Healthy* magazine and *Spa World*. She has contributed to numerous other publications and is the face behind such bestselling books and DVDs as *Fight Fat, Fight Fatigue*; *Energy Makeover*;

The Sugar Addict's Diet and *Nicki Waterman's Flat Stomach Plan*. Nicki is also the fitness consultant and choreographer for the *Strictly Come Dancersize* DVDs and frequently appears on *GMTV* and *Britain's Next Top Model*. She holds Fitness For Industry, ACE (American Council of Exercise) and Focus Training advanced certificates and is an accredited YMCA Personal Trainer. Her clients include many celebrities, our very own Denise Van Outen among them.

Working with Denise is Sam Mann, a highly respected journalist in the celebrity field, not only in print but also in TV and radio. A regular contributor to some of the biggest publications in the UK, Sam wrote a weekly column in the *Daily Mirror* for over five years and frequently appears on TV shows including ITV's *This Morning*. Over the last ten years Sam has interviewed everyone in the music industry, from McCartney to Madonna, not to mention an impressive list of big screen stars. Will Smith, Dustin Hoffman and Angelina Jolie are all up there on Sam's list of favourite interviewees, but top of the list, of course, is her friend Denise. Their great friendship has allowed Sam to gain a real insight into the journey Denise undertook throughout her pregnancy.

Chapter One

Get Ready, Get Set...

Me and My Fertility

What's going on in your body?

Not much yet – but watch this space!

My Diary

As my good friends enthused about their exciting plans – a family camping trip, teddy bear's picnic and kiddies' birthday parties – I felt miserable. Every year I get together with a couple of old girlfriends from my *Big Breakfast* days, to catch up on everything that's been happening in our lives. I always look forward to it so much, loving nothing more than a good gossip with the girls.

These days, Cockney Vik was a doting mum to her daughter Annabel, and Anna had two adorable boys and was now pregnant with her third. As for me, I'd just told them I'd landed a new job working alongside my old *BB* sidekick Johnny Vaughn on the Capital Radio Breakfast Show. But instead of feeling excited and proud as I normally would about my work achievements, I felt embarrassed. Was this all I had to offer? Was I destined to work my life away?

That was when I realised things had to change.

Don't get me wrong, I know I'm extremely lucky to have had such amazing opportunities and to get paid for doing the things I'm so passionate about, but hearing my friends talk about their children just made me feel like there was a huge gaping hole in my life. Over the last couple of years I'd spent time living the single life in Los Angeles, mending my broken heart after losing my beloved Nan, and facing up to yet another failed romance. (When he told me on our first date he was in therapy for commitment issues, I should have ran a mile – but alas, we always think we'll be the one to change them, don't we, girls?) I'd also been working harder than I'd ever worked in my life, and I consider myself to be a grafter. I was hosting a show called *Grease Is the Word* for the American TV network NBC, which was keeping me busy enough, when I received a call from Andrew Lloyd Webber's office offering me a job I couldn't refuse. A few weeks later I found myself flying back to the UK each week to sit on the judging panel for *Any Dream Will Do*, the BBC series in which we searched to find a new star for Andrew Lloyd Webber's musical *Joseph and the Amazing Technicolour Dreamcoat*.

Both were fantastic experiences and I loved working with so many talented people (not to mention getting to know a certain cutie who was one of the contestants on *Any Dream Will Do!*), but I can't say I missed the weekly transatlantic flights when both shows came to an end. Once my time at NBC had finished, I moved back to London and settled into my new theatre role, playing Maureen in the West End musical *Rent*.

I had been back in London for a matter of days when Lee Mead, the handsome chap who been the winner of *Any Dream Will Do*, called to ask me out on a date… and the rest, as they say, is history. So that night when I was sitting with my *Big Breakfast* pals feeling a little sorry for myself, there was at least a glimmer of hope. Perhaps the future wasn't going to be *all* about work. I now had a lovely new boyfriend and our relationship was going extremely well.

However, a couple of weeks after my girly get-together I began my new job at Capital Radio and before long my schedule was as busy as ever. Not only was I getting up at a quarter past four every morning but I was also filming until ten o'clock each evening. I was now a panellist on the BBC show *I'd Do Anything*, searching for someone to play Oliver in the stage show of the same name, as well as simultaneously hosting *Hairspray: The School Musical* for Sky1.

My ridiculous hours and lack of sleep left me exhausted. It all came to a head just a week before I turned thirty-four. I felt as though I was falling apart and began to panic. For my own peace of mind I booked myself a full-body medical MOT. I had my breasts checked (by a doctor, not Lee), all my moles examined, and I was also offered a fertility test, which rather took me by surprise. It seemed unnecessary so I declined it at first, but the doctor insisted it would be good to put my mind at rest. As it all came as part of the package, I decided to go for it, telling myself that at least the doctor could give me advice in the unlikely event there was something wrong.

I wasn't remotely expecting anything abnormal to show up, but it turned out I was in for a bit of a shock. The doctor told me my ovarian egg reserve was low for someone my age. Worryingly, this meant it could take me a couple of years to get pregnant. On the plus side, thanks to the doctor's persistence, at least I knew where I stood.

I went home straight away and called my mum to tell her how it had gone. Of course she wasn't expecting me to have a fertility test so was shocked when I explained what had happened. I was trying desperately not to sound too upset, but mums can always tell. She was quick to reassure me that everything would be OK and told me I needed to talk it through with Lee. We said our goodbyes and I was about to hang up when I realised she hadn't put the receiver down properly. Without intending to, I overheard her repeating our conversation to my dad, who said he hoped I wasn't going to miss out on motherhood and that he had worried that something like this would happen. It upset me even more to hear him so concerned – he knew that becoming a mother was always such a big part of my plan for the future.

As soon as Lee arrived home I explained everything the doctor had said. He was very understanding and I didn't detect an ounce of panic (if it was a cover-up, he deserved an Oscar for his performance). He told me there was only one thing to do: crack on with it! He did have one condition, though, which was that we got married first. That was fine with me but I had one condition of my own: that he take a break from the *Joseph* loincloth and wear a nice morning suit for our big day!

Lee's reaction was such a relief as most of the guys I had dated in the past would have run a mile. We had spoken really early on in our relationship about how much we both wanted children and his mum had even told me that his main aim in life had always been to meet the right girl, settle down and start a family. I was truly lucky.

However, I still needed to actually fall pregnant. After explaining what a low egg reserve meant, the doctor had advised me that it would require a complete change of lifestyle on my part if I wanted to increase my chances of conception. My schedule was hectic and at the time I was averaging between four and five hours of sleep a night. I was working flat out all day, every day, often without a single break. I'd noticed the lack of daylight in my life had started to affect my mood and I was the closest I'd ever come to feeling depressed. My diet was seriously suffering, too. Most mornings I'd be in such a rush that I'd skip breakfast and the first seven hours of my day would be fuelled by copious amounts of caffeine. With my radio show over, I'd whizz across London to the TV studio to start my day of filming. That'd be when I'd eat my first meal of the day, often something quick and easy like a croissant from the canteen or a slice of toast with jam. When my energy levels dipped during the day I'd reach for a can of Coke to pep me up. If I was lucky enough to get a late lunch I'd grab a chicken salad sandwich or, on the rare occasion I'd have more than thirty minutes to eat, I'd indulge in a jacket potato loaded with beans and cheese. My afternoons unfortunately didn't get any healthier, as anyone who has ever worked on or visited a TV film set will know that the chocolate is dished out like it's going out of fashion.

With the chocolate, caffeine and adrenaline still rushing through my system I'd arrive home late, still buzzing. I'd eventually drift off to sleep at midnight for four hours of precious shut-eye before my day would begin all over again.

After much soul-searching there was no denying that it was my job at Capital Radio that was affecting me the most. The incredibly early starts meant I was constantly shattered. I decided to approach my boss. Luckily he was very gracious and understood that despite still having six months to run on my contract I needed to leave for health reasons. It was a big decision to go but the right one for me.

My next step was to contact my good friend, the fitness expert Nicki Waterman. I've had Nicki's number on speed dial for the last ten years and whenever I have needed to get fit for my West End shows she's helped me enormously. Having Nicki there to motivate and inspire me was crucial to getting me back on track quickly.

But of course, getting physically fit was only half the challenge. I desperately needed to change my diet and could think of no one better to help me do that than Nicki's pal and partner-in-crime, the nutritionist Amanda Ursell. I knew that with their expert advice behind me I was putting myself in the best possible position to fall pregnant.

I was an Essex girl on a mission.

Now for the Experts...

Exercise and fertility

So, you and your partner have finally made the decision to try to conceive. Your mind may be racing with all the things you've heard about exercise when you're trying for a baby – what you should do; what you shouldn't do; can exercise actually help you get pregnant in the first place? Here's what you should know.

Does exercise aid fertility?

Yes. When done in moderation and after discussion with your doctor, exercise can help in your quest to get pregnant. The key is that word 'moderation' – you don't want to push yourself too far. Some female athletes, for example, exercise so much that they actually stop menstruation, which would of course hinder their ability to conceive. So don't go for the burn and don't exercise to exhaustion. A good rule of thumb is to slow down if you can't comfortably carry on a conversation while moving.

How does exercise help you fall pregnant?

Exercise aids fertility in a number of ways. First of all, it can be difficult for you to become pregnant if you are overweight, as excess body fat can interfere with your menstrual cycle. Therefore, for the same reason that you don't want to be underweight when you begin attempting to conceive, you don't want to be overweight either (see pages 22–23 for more information on the recommended Body Mass Index). Exercise, combined with a good diet, can help you maintain a healthy body weight, which in turn helps you achieve pregnancy.

Not only that, but a fit body can also help to make your sex life more enjoyable, resulting in stronger orgasms. This is also believed to help with conception, as the uterus will 'dip down' during an orgasm and help the semen make its way up into the uterus. Naturally a healthy body will also make a stronger environment for a baby to grow and help with eventual labour.

There is also another, less direct, way in which exercise influences conception. A good workout releases hormone-like chemicals called *endorphins* into your body. Put simply, endorphins make you happy. The happier you are, the more likely you are to be relaxed and in the mood for sex. Sounds silly? It's not. Even mild depression can hinder your chances of becoming pregnant, and exercise can be an effective treatment for this. Working out, therefore, can help reduce stress and lead to a better night's sleep – again an essential part of maintaining a healthy lifestyle, as Denise found to her cost when she was doing her radio breakfast show. A well-rested body can work on healing itself while you sleep and will maximise the nutrients found in a healthy diet.

But I've heard that exercise can hurt my chances of getting pregnant!

It's pretty unlikely that mild to moderate exercise will hinder your ability to conceive. However, the definition of moderate exercise varies from person to person, so if you are trying but not managing to fall pregnant you may want to take a brief hiatus from the gym to rule out its involvement in the delay. Ultimately, this is why it's important to discuss your exercise regime with your doctor while you're trying to conceive.

Nicki's advice

If you plan to get pregnant, get as fit as you possibly can first. However, when actually trying to conceive, take exercise down to what you'd do if you were pregnant – i.e. no more than half an hour a day. If you're pregnant and you're only going to do one thing, make it pelvic floor exercises (see page 51).
In a nutshell: pregnancy is no excuse to put your feet up.

Good ways to exercise when pregnant or trying for a baby

Swimming

Swimming is a gentle but effective workout that you can easily continue throughout your pregnancy. Swimming is good for cardiovascular function and uses many different muscle groups, particularly in your arms and legs. At the same time it's a low-impact sport that's easy to vary in terms of intensity. Importantly, the water offers good support to pregnant women, putting less gravitational strain on the joints and making the risk of injury very low. The blissful sense of weightlessness is a welcome relief in those later, heavy months, and the water also stops you from overheating during your workout. For more on swimming and aqua-aerobics, see pages 116–18.

Water aerobics

If the idea of a watery workout appeals but you find it difficult to motivate yourself to exercise alone, why not try an aqua-aerobics or aqua-exercise class? Aqua-aerobics is focused more on fat burning, while aqua-exercise is aimed at improving muscle tone, strength and mobility. Water is ideal for pregnancy training, as it provides resistance without exposing you to the high-impact pounding that can be dangerous while pregnant. You don't even need to be able to swim to participate in these workouts as many moves are performed in waist- or chest-high water.

Walking

The best thing about walking is that it's so easy to fit into your normal life. A good brisk walk for about thirty minutes will also get your heart going – though if you're not used to the exercise then start off with shorter walks and build up with a few extra minutes each time. If you want to be a bit more serious about it and work out your arms too, you could try Nordic walking, using supportive poles to pump your arms as you walk.

Low-impact aerobic classes or exercise DVDs

Whether you're someone who enjoys the sociable aspect of an aerobics class down at your local gym or whether you prefer to work out in the privacy of your own home, there is a class or a DVD out there that will suit you.

Cycling

As long as you stick to normal cycle paths and roads, cycling is a great low-impact workout that you can continue during pregnancy if you're careful. However, do bear in mind it isn't as low-risk as walking or swimming, as there is always the chance that you could fall off your bike. Cycling off-road can often be more physically demanding and you should leave that to others once you're pregnant due to the higher likelihood of taking a tumble.

Yoga and pilates

Yoga and pilates are great for building up muscle tone, developing flexibility and for helping you relax. Both also have the advantage that you can later move on to pregnancy-specific courses and exercises. However, do be aware that some types of yoga are very strenuous and not suited to women who are trying to fall pregnant (see pages 100–1 for more on different types of yoga).

Nutrition and fertility

Denise was absolutely right to start thinking about her diet as soon as she made the momentous decision to create new life.

For many women, in fact about half, pregnancy is not planned and they don't have the opportunity to get their nutritional health in good shape beforehand. But that means fifty per cent do, and if you are one of those reading this now, that's great news – because what you eat around the time of conception can have an effect not just on the development of the baby in your tummy, but also, somewhat remarkably, on its health well into adult life too.

If this sounds a bit far-fetched, then consider this. Within just ten short weeks of the sperm and egg colliding with each other in your fallopian tubes, these two cells will have replicated some six billion times. Yes, *six billion*.

In fact, within three weeks of the single sperm and egg coming together it is incredible to think that already the development of a heart, brain, spinal cord and blood vessels has already got underway.

These rapidly dividing cells need a great supply of nutrients for the process to proceed optimally. Given that you will not know for sure which month you will conceive, the best advice is to make sure that you are giving your body these nutrients every day from the moment you decide that you want to have a baby.

Any irregular eating patterns like Denise's have to stop. Regular, healthy and balanced meals are crucial from now on. Surviving on chocolate and snatched sandwiches, skipping meals and keeping energy levels up with caffeine really can lower your chances of conceiving, and if you do manage to fall pregnant, it will affect your baby's very earliest development. This means that if your lifestyle makes it easy to opt for a poor diet then you must, as Denise did, sort out your priorities and put food high up on the list of things to fix.

So, first things first. If you have been on a perennial weight-loss plan then stop following it right away. Ditto if you've been cutting your calories to shape up for an upcoming event like a party or a beach holiday. If you have been missing breakfast, make sure you find time to have it. And if you survive on junk, sweets, crisps, biscuits and fast food, it is time to draw the line and swap them for nutrient-packed alternatives. You wouldn't feed your baby a burger and fries followed by a coffee once it is born, so why feed it this kind of food when it is developing in your tummy?

What you should be eating when pregnant or trying for a baby

For information on what you should be avoiding eating when trying for a baby and during pregnancy, please see Chapter Four. In the meantime, these are the things you *should* be consuming to maximise your health:

Folic acid

As soon as you decide to try for a baby, go straight to the nearest pharmacy and invest in folic acid supplements. Folic acid is a member of the B vitamin family and you need to take 400 micrograms of this nutrient every day prior to conception and in the first twelve weeks of your baby's development. Studies have shown this will significantly decrease the chances of your baby being born with spina bifida, a challenging condition to live with that affects the spinal cord.

We can get folic acid in foods such as black-eyed beans, beetroot and oranges, but even a well-balanced diet usually only provides 200 micrograms a day. Using supplements boosts your intake to the protective level needed.

Breakfast

You will need to start having three regular meals a day. This means no more skipping breakfast – and no more muffins and croissants. They may have kept you going in your young, free and single days, but when you are planning the biggest creative feat of your life, you should avoid the largely empty calories these types of foods provide.

What you need are foods that are packed with vitamins and minerals, and those that contain useful amounts of protein and slow-release energy to keep you going and keep cravings for unhealthy snacks at bay.

Take a leaf out of Denise's book and make some porridge, or opt for nutritious ready-to-eat breakfast cereals (e.g. Oatibix or Weetabix) or sugar-free muesli. Eat them with skimmed or semi-skimmed milk and preferably with some fruit too.

Other good options include hard-boiled eggs, scrambled eggs or omelette. Eggs need to be well-cooked to avoid any potential problems with the food poisoning bug salmonella.

Ten quick nutrient-packed snacks

- Handful of almonds
- A banana and an oatcake
- Hummus on a couple of crispbreads
- Apple with peanut butter on a slice of toast
- A fresh fruit salad with fromage frais
- 0% or 2% fat Greek yoghurt with berries
- A mini Babybel cheese with some grapes
- A handful of chopped dried apricots with five chopped cashew nuts
- Ricotta cheese and celery with some breadsticks
- A slice of wholemeal toast with dark chocolate spread and some strawberries

Lunch

A sustaining and healthy lunch could be anything from a tortilla wrap filled with lean roast chicken and salad with some reduced-fat salad cream to keep it moist and tasty, to a pitta bread stuffed with hummus and salad, or a lean roast beef sandwich on granary bread with tomatoes and cucumber. All options can be followed by a yoghurt and fruit.

Dinner

A lean steak; some baked salmon; a stir-fry using soya beans or tofu or lean turkey or pork; a lean roast dinner with lots of vegetables and a baked potato… all are wholesome, nutrient-rich dinners that are great to tuck into.

Vitamin and mineral checklist

Vitamins

Folic acid should be covered by your 400-microgram daily supplement, but it is also important to continue eating foods that are rich in this essential nutrient.

You can get it from: fortified breakfast cereals (check the nutrition label), black-eyed beans, Brussels sprouts, peanuts, spinach, broccoli, chickpeas, avocados, oranges, peanut butter, baked beans, wholegrain bread.

Note: steam vegetables lightly because heat destroys folic acid.

Vitamin B1 ensures that energy contained in the foods we ingest is transported to each cell in your body and that of your developing baby. You could be deficient in this vitamin if you have been dieting or eating badly, so make sure that you start topping up as quickly as you can. You will also need a little more B1 in the last three months of pregnancy.

You can get it from: yeast extracts (e.g. Marmite), peas, oranges, fortified breakfast cereals, boiled potatoes, pork, eggs, wholegrain cereals (e.g. brown pasta and wholegrain bread). Most foods on a healthy eating diet provide you with B1.

Vitamin B2 levels need to go up slightly when pregnant. Like B1, B2 is also important for helping our body to release and use energy from the foods we eat. If you have been on a weight-reducing diet in the past (and who hasn't?), the chances are that your B2 levels could be below par and need a boost. Prior to pregnancy, women need 1.1 mg of B2, and once pregnant this rises to 1.4 mg daily.

You can get it from: dairy foods such as milk (a pint of skimmed milk will cover your daily needs), along with yoghurts, fortified cereals, eggs, lean beef, chicken and, again, yeast extract.

Niacin is yet another B vitamin that helps turn food energy into a form our cells can use. Although niacin is found in lots of foods and women in the UK tend to get enough, it is wise to ensure that you eat the following regularly.

You can get it from: lean meats such as beef, pork, chicken or turkey, wheatgerm, Cheddar cheese, wholegrain cereals (e.g. wholemeal bread), cod and eggs. Peanuts and fortified breakfast cereals are also good for niacin.

Vitamin B6 is another crucial pregnancy B vitamin and, although needs don't officially rise when pregnant, some women do not hit the 1.2 mg daily target in the first place. It is therefore worth checking that you are including some of the foods below in your diet to make sure you get sufficient quantities.

You can get it from: wheatgerm, cod, turkey, beef, bananas, Brussels sprouts, cabbage and mangos, along with fortified breakfast cereals, steamed salmon, canned tuna and avocados.

Vitamin B12 is hard to be deficient in unless you are vegan because it is found in all protein-based foods from animal sources. Women need 1.5 micrograms daily and this doesn't increase in pregnancy. It's used to make healthy nerves and to aid growth.

You can get it from: all meats and fish, eggs, milk and fortified breakfast cereals.

Vitamin C is important for healthy immunity and to keep our gums and skin in good condition, as well as being important for improving the absorption of iron from plant-based foods. Needs increase from 40 mg daily to 50 mg when pregnant. Most women get around 60 mg a day and so should be OK, but if you are having your 'five a day' of fruits and vegetables, you are probably getting more.

You can get it from: all citrus fruits such as oranges and grapefruit, papaya, guava, blackcurrants and other berries like strawberries. Also peppers, broccoli, kiwi fruits, cabbage and cauliflower.

Vitamin A is important for the growth of your baby, particularly in the first three months. While a low level of vitamin A in pregnant women's blood is linked with retardation of growth, low birth weight and premature birth, women in the UK get on average almost 1500 micrograms daily, which is just over double the 700 micrograms requirement in pregnancy.

However, while it's important to receive sufficient levels of vitamin A during pregnancy, having *excess* amounts can be even more of a problem. This is something which must be avoided because too much (8,000 to 10,000 micrograms daily) may cause birth defects. Therefore, because liver is a very rich source of vitamin A, it is advised that liver and foods made from it (like liver patés) are avoided during pregnancy, along with fish oil supplements that are also high in vitamin A.

Incidentally, this is also why it is important not to supplement with any multivitamins that are not recommended by your doctor or have not been specifically designed for pregnant women.

You can get it from: butter and margarine, eggs, whole milk – all of which contain safe levels of vitamin A. It is also found in oily fish, though pregnant women should have no more than one serving of oily fish a week.

Vitamin D is the so-called 'sunshine' vitamin, required to help our bodies absorb the bone-building mineral calcium. Although in theory women should make enough vitamin D through the action of sunlight on our skin, converting 'pro-vitamin D' into the active form during the months of March to September in the UK, the fact remains that most of us don't seem to manage this. There are few foods rich in this vitamin and so most women probably need to take a 10-microgram supplement daily to meet needs.

You can get it from: oily fish like herrings, mackerel, sardines, trout and salmon – but remember, you are only supposed to have one serving a week when pregnant. Other foods containing small amounts of vitamin D include margarine and eggs.

Minerals

The good news about minerals is that they don't get destroyed through cooking but, on the other hand, they can sometimes be tricky to absorb – though you shouldn't worry if you are eating a healthy, balanced diet. There are numerous different minerals but the four main ones that are extra-important for pregnancy are as follows.

Magnesium is needed for strong bones and teeth but also, importantly, it seems that this mineral is vital for supporting the very rapid division of cells that takes place just after conception. Research has revealed that poor intakes are associated with low birth weights, which themselves lead to complications such as an increased risk of infant ill-health generally, including damage to the brain and nervous system, and even loss of life.

The recommended intake each day for magnesium is 270 mg. The reason we need to take particular care is because food surveys reveal that, on average, women only get 237 mg daily. This means that quite a lot of us need to up our intakes, especially when planning a pregnancy.

You can get it from: wholegrain cereals, wholemeal and granary breads, rye crispbreads, sunflower and pumpkin seeds, nuts, peanut butter, pilchards, lentils and spinach.

Calcium is vital for your own bones to remain strong and for the developing bones of your baby in the womb. It seems that your baby probably takes what it needs at your expense, so having enough calcium in your diet while pregnant is essential for your own long-term health.

Although the recommended amount of 700 mg a day remains the same when you are pregnant, the fact is that the average British woman aged sixteen to thirty-four has an intake that falls below this. If you are in this category, it means that you could start your pregnancy behind the game.

You can get it from: milk (skimmed is a little better than whole and semi-skimmed), yoghurt, fortified soya milk, steamed tofu, sesame seeds, canned sardines (eaten with the bones), dried figs, green beans and other dark green vegetables. Cheese is also great for calcium.

Zinc is needed to help cells to replicate, which makes it particularly important in the first few weeks and months of pregnancy. If you start off with poor zinc reserves, it can affect the development of your baby's brain and central nervous system.

Women who are demi- or completely vegetarian can have less than optimal zinc levels, along with women who have taken the contraceptive pill for a long time and those who do a lot of hard fitness training. Target intakes are 7 mg a day for all women. Eating a well-balanced diet should meet these needs.

You can get it from: wheatgerm, pumpkin seeds, lean red meats, canned crab, sardines canned in oil.

Iron is essential for the cells in our bodies to get sufficient oxygen, because iron helps to make the oxygen-carrying haemoglobin in our blood.

During pregnancy our iron needs do not increase, partly because we stop menstruation which saves quite a bit of iron that is usually lost through blood, and partly because our bodies seem to switch on mechanisms to help us absorb more than usual from our regular foods.

The problem is that around forty per cent of women aged eighteen to thirty-four in the UK do not get enough of this mineral in the first place. If you don't have enough during pregnancy, your body appears to make sure that your baby does not go short, by increasing the amounts passing through the placenta. However, this can leave you feeling tired and stressed, with poor concentration and low resistance to infections. If you develop full-blown iron-deficiency anaemia, you could end up with a greater risk of your baby arriving early and having a low birth weight as a result.

You can get it from: animal-derived foods like lean red meats, oily fish such as sardines and game meats (e.g. venison). It is well absorbed from these foods. You also get iron from plant foods such as dried apricots, fortified breakfast cereals, sesame seeds, cashew nuts and peanuts. It is believed that the tannin in tea reduces our ability to absorb iron from these foods (so avoid drinking tea with your meals if you are at risk of iron deficiency), while eating vitamin C-rich foods like citrus fruits and fruit juices enhances it.

A word on weight

Being underweight, which means having a Body Mass Index (see box opposite) of less than 20, can lead to your periods stopping, which of course makes conception next to impossible. Also, underweight mothers are more likely to have babies born with a low birth weight. This is probably a reflection of a general poor diet in the mother rather than a direct causal relation, but whatever the reason, it is a bad idea to be too light when trying to have a baby if you can avoid it.

Women with a BMI of over 30, on the other hand, will also find it harder to conceive and, if they do, they are more likely to suffer problems such as raised blood pressure, pregnancy diabetes and pre-eclampsia, which can be dangerous to both mother and baby. According to recent figures, about half of women of childbearing age are either overweight (with a BMI of 25 to 29.9) or obese (with a BMI of 30 or above), and approximately sixteen per cent of women in England are obese from the start of pregnancy.

A BMI of 23 to 24 seems to be optimal for fertility and your baby's ultimate birth weight. The best way to gain weight as well as shedding it is by combining a balanced diet with regular exercise. You should also aim to take a daily vitamin and mineral supplement (with fifty to seventy per cent of the RDA of each included) and to get to your target weight about two to three months before starting to try for your baby. Trying to get your BMI into the normal range is important if you are planning a healthy pregnancy.

How to calculate your BMI

Write down your weight in kilograms and divide it by the square of your height in metres. (If you want to use Imperial measures, take your weight in pounds, multiply it by 703, then divide that by your height in inches squared.)

So a woman who is 1.65 m (approx 5' 5" or 65 in) tall and weighs 60 kg (approx 9½ stone or 133 lb), would calculate her BMI as follows:

60 ÷ (1.65 x 1.65 = 2.72) = 22

Chapter Two

Go!

Conception

What's going on in your body?

You may not realise this, but the first two weeks of your pregnancy occur before conception takes place! This is because the forty weeks of pregnancy are timed from the first day of your last menstrual period, not from conception. So what is called 'four weeks' pregnant' is actually about two weeks from conception.

During your last period, the lining of your uterus would have thickened up as usual to receive a fertilised egg, while several eggs were busy maturing in your ovaries. Once they are released, the eggs live for about twelve to twenty-four hours as they make their way down your Fallopian tube. If conception is to take place, an egg must be fertilised within this time by a single plucky sperm – though be aware that sperm can live for several days inside a woman's body (and a man can release 300 million sperm in one ejaculation!). So if that sperm has wriggled his way up that Fallopian tube when that egg is still hanging around – bingo! Congratulations, you're pregnant…

My Diary

With my job at Capital Radio behind me, I used the extra hours in my day to catch up on some of the sleep I'd missed out on over the past six months and to start my new fitness regime under Nicki's guidance. We regularly met up on Hampstead Heath for walks and built up to gentle runs. Bit by bit, I was starting to feel like my old self again.

Despite my early enthusiasm, Nicki suggested that I find another incentive to keep up the exercise. She explained that it's pretty easy to motivate yourself when the sun is shining, but when it's cold and raining you need an extra goal to get you out of the door. Of course I wanted to be as healthy as possible to improve my fertility so was convinced I'd be totally committed, but a short-term goal to focus on couldn't harm.

Having witnessed the dedication and training my good mate David Walliams put into his cross-Channel swim for Sport Relief, I remember thinking that I'd love to set myself a similar physical challenge one day (however not one that involved slipping on a pair of Speedos and greasing up with goose fat). So with Nicki's advice ringing in my ears, I made a mental decision there and then to sign up for the London Marathon.

After we'd finished our training session I dashed home to look into registering online. I'd literally just sat down at the computer when my mobile rang. I was surprised to hear Gary Barlow's voice on the other end and intrigued when he said he had a proposition for me. This was it, I was about to become the first female member of Take That! Alas, my moment of excitement was short-lived, as sadly he had no intention of inviting me to join the fab four (now five, of course). Instead he asked if I fancied joining him in climbing a mountain. Not your average Saturday afternoon request! He went on to explain he was rounding up a team of celebrities to climb Mount Kilimanjaro in Africa in aid of Comic Relief. He'd barely paused for breath when I said I'd love to do it. He chuckled at my enthusiasm before explaining it wasn't something to be taken lightly. Kili is the tallest mountain in Africa, over fifteen thousand feet above sea level. People have died while attempting to reach the top (a little different from Hampstead Heath then). He suggested I do some research before I said yes, to make sure I knew what I was getting into, but I'd already made up my mind. I was going to be part of his team.

Nicki couldn't believe it when I called to tell her what had just happened – it was obviously meant to be, following our conversation earlier that day. She stressed how important it was not to rush into my training and that the best way to build up my fitness was to do so gradually otherwise I'd be putting my body under stress once again, which of course would be bad news for my fertility. We gently built up the intensity of our workouts and before long my main focus was the climb.

Every press interview I did to promote Comic Relief had a similar theme: after a couple of questions about the cause, the usual barrage of enquiries would follow about my relationship with Lee and when we were going to start a family. I'd cobble together a woolly answer, all the while wondering whether I could actually conceive. During that same period there also appeared to be some kind of mini baby boom among my friends and colleagues. There seemed to be a new 'OMG I'm pregnant!' announcement every day. Of course I was overjoyed for every one of them, yet each one also left me feeling a bit strange, given the dark cloud I had hanging over my own fertility. I'm sure any woman who has been told she has low fertility or has been trying to conceive for a while will know how I felt. It was as if Mother Nature was conspiring against me.

I didn't confide in anyone about how I was feeling and I didn't even want Lee to see how it was affecting me, but I had plenty of moments when I'd be home alone pottering around my flat worrying about what we'd do if we couldn't have children. I'd remember the tearful conversations I had with one of my best friends when she was undergoing IVF and the strain it had put on her otherwise stable relationship. I wondered how Lee and I would cope if we had to go down the same route. I'd also often wake up super-early and lie there next to Lee for hours, playing everything through in my mind. I know, as the saying goes, that there's no use worrying about what hasn't happened yet, but I couldn't help it.

My exercise became an escape for me and Nicki was surprised by how quickly I had become almost addicted to it. I'd ring her when it was awful weather outside to tell her I still wanted to meet up. As I trained regularly I could feel myself getting fitter; I was sleeping better; I was much happier in myself; and I was getting my sparkle back. I hadn't realised until then that I'd been avoiding seeing my friends, not only because I was so busy but because I didn't feel like I had anything to talk about apart from what I was working on. I was also craving healthier food, which made it easy for me to stick to Amanda's dietary guidelines, and I had a regular pattern when it came to my trips to the loo for the first time in ages (hooray, no need for the prunes any more!). Those days of caffeine and chocolate were starting to feel like a lifetime ago.

My hard work with Nicki paid off and on 7 March 2009, along with my celebrity team-mates, I made it to the top of Mount Kilimanjaro. The whole experience blew me away and I can't

recommend doing something similar highly enough – though
obviously not everyone will be lucky or mad enough to climb
a mountain! But whatever your physical goal, pushing yourself
beyond what you think you are capable of is an exhilarating feeling.
It was without doubt the most challenging and rewarding thing
I'd ever done and not only gave me an experience I'll never forget
but also symbolised my life turning around 180 degrees from how
it had been a few months before, when I was eating unhealthily,
barely seeing the sunshine and fending off depression.

I now had my healthy lifestyle firmly in place and wanted to turn
my full attention to getting up the duff but, as per Lee's request
(demand, more like!), I had one major thing to sort out first. So in
April 2009, in a wonderful ceremony on a beach in the Seychelles
with my family and close friends there to celebrate with me, I was
overjoyed to become Mrs Mead. It was everything I had dreamed
of and more. And of course, no sooner had we said good night to
the last guests at the reception than we got cracking with the task in
hand. Happy days.

I was both excited and relaxed about it at first but our busy
schedules soon began to create problems. Lee was in New York
attending an acting course while I was busy working on various
projects in London. When I had time I'd spend a fortune clocking
up the air miles trying to coordinate being with my man when I
thought I was ovulating. And let me tell you, discovering when
ovulation was occurring was a mission in itself. One friend
informed me I should be able to 'feel' when my eggs were being
released, another said my temperature would go up slightly and
I should then perform the 'mucus test'. This involved sticking my
hand right down below to collect some discharge, then testing the
consistency between my index finger and thumb to determine how

sticky it was. The stickier the better as it's a good indication that ovulation is taking place. I must admit to having a few moments of disbelief when trying this one out. I even bought those little sticks you pee on from the chemist too. It was all a bit confusing to be honest, but we kept on trying everything regardless.

As Lee returned from New York, I had to move up to Edinburgh for a four-week stint at the Edinburgh Festival. By this point it seemed like everything was conspiring against us. I was performing a one-woman show every day and with the physical and mental exertion I was in bed, knackered, by ten o'clock every night. I put my tiredness down to the adrenaline of being on stage and the busy year I'd had, so I was looking forward to spending some quality time with my new husband when I got home.

When I got back to London it was time to let my hair down with a much-needed girly barbecue with Anna and Cockney Vik, but after a few sips of wine I felt quite drunk. This was completely out of character for me as I'm usually the last one standing. It was only when Anna asked me if there was a chance that I could be pregnant that the penny dropped. Perhaps that was the reason why I'd been feeling so tired? Come to think of it I had eaten the same thing for lunch every day while I was up in Edinburgh – a Cheddar cheese baguette. Perhaps I was experiencing my first craving?

I stumbled home to Lee and explained what had happened. For some reason, despite the transatlantic trips in conjunction with my ovarian calendar, the healthy lifestyle, and the great deal of trying I'd made him do (it's not all bad, this baby-making lark), Lee thought it was highly unlikely I was pregnant and I was probably just under the weather. He persuaded me to save the only pregnancy test we had left in my top drawer – not because it cost ten pounds and he's a skinflint, but because buying the test itself without anyone seeing you is a real mission when you're in the public eye. Lee thought that an early night was probably all I needed to feel like myself again. We curled up in bed and I felt a bit silly that I'd even allowed myself to think I could be pregnant.

At four o'clock in the morning I sat bolt upright in bed and I swear I could feel my hormones racing around my body. I shook Lee awake and, bless him, he stumbled out of bed and stood by me as I opened our last pregnancy test with my fingers trembling. I did a wee and waited those three minutes that seem more like hours. I looked down to see two pink lines and shrieked with delight.

I – we – were finally pregnant.

Now for the Experts...

Starting exercising and staying motivated

As we saw in the previous chapter, there's plenty of evidence that couples who are generally fit and healthy will find it easier to conceive and maintain a pregnancy beyond its early stages. (This advice does not just apply to women, by the way – it's good for men to look at their lifestyle when thinking of starting a family. Lee started going to the gym too when he and Denise were trying to conceive!)

It's also true that if you're used to regular exercise before you conceive then it will be easier for you to maintain a fitness regime throughout your pregnancy. Not only will this help you adjust to the huge physical and even emotional changes you'll experience and help ease the discomforts pregnancy can bring, but also good stamina, flexibility and controlled breathing can make all the difference during labour itself.

If you're not used to exercising then introduce it slowly, keeping your aims within easy reach and building up the number, length and intensity of your exercise sessions each week. You should aim to get at least four workouts of twenty minutes each per week and ideally four to five sessions of thirty to forty minutes, working up a slight sweat. It's a good idea to vary the type and intensity of workouts. Whatever form of exercise you do, remember to leave time to warm up beforehand, and stretch and cool down afterwards.

Ten motivational exercise tips that won't let you down

1 **Set yourself a goal.** You might not be able to climb Mount Kilimanjaro like Denise, but could you train for a swimathon or a five-kilometre charity run in your local park? Even a small regular goal like aiming to take the stairs rather than the lift at every opportunity, or walking to work rather than taking the bus, will help raise your fitness levels.

2 **Write it down.** When you make a commitment on paper to work out, you're more likely to do so. Write it in your daily appointment book – and then keep that appointment.

3 **Beat inertia.** When you come home from work and haven't had a chance to exercise yet, don't slump on the sofa. Slip on some trainers and get out there, even if it's only for a ten-minute walk.

4 **Get obligated.** Commit to someone else. You will motivate each other to make time for fitness.

5 **Know your fitness personality.** Are you a morning or night person? An outdoor or indoor person? A social person or a loner? Do you love or hate loud music? Do you need an instructor to motivate you? Or do you prefer to work out using a machine? Once you have determined your fitness 'personality', it will be easier for you to select a programme that you will stick with.

6 **Reward yourself.** Choose a non-calorific reward like a massage or a facial every time you fulfil your weekly workout goals.

7 **Keep it realistic.** Recognise that you have time restrictions and, if you are already pregnant, that you won't be able to do as much as you could pre-pregnancy. Working out less intensively but consistently will give you better results.

8 **Wear what works.** Form-fitting, fun colours, great fashion – all can be motivators. If you like what you're wearing, you may want to wear it more often. For some people it's baggy track-pants and an old T-shirt. Find out what works for you.

9 **Get a pedometer for the daytime.** Current thinking suggests ten thousand steps per day are needed for good health. Try walking whenever you can in your day – you will be further motivated as you see the steps clock up!

10 **Set the score.** The wrong music can drag your routine down. Download some upbeat music on to your iPod or mp3 player.

Nutrition in early pregnancy

As we mentioned in Chapter One, folic acid is crucial in the early stages of pregnancy, so if your positive test is a shock and not planned, do start taking it as soon as you realise that you have conceived.

There is still time to get the rest of your diet in hand, too. From the moment you know you're pregnant, dump the junk, cut out the booze and caffeine, and start to eat regularly and healthily as outlined in Chapter One.

In the first thirteen weeks of pregnancy, an extraordinary feat of reproduction is going on inside your body. Your baby, which started as two cells, is growing at an incredible rate, developing a heart, blood vessels, brain and spinal cord, sprouting arms and legs, fingers and toes, eyes and ears... And here is the thing: *you* are the sole provider of nutrients to enable the division of cells to create all these amazing organs and body parts. When you grasp this, it makes it a lot easier to see why good nutrition is so crucial.

Between weeks three to eight is the time when your developing baby is most at risk of so-called *environmental sensitivity.* Any setbacks like exposure to cigarette smoke or drugs, maternal infections or poor nutrition at this vulnerable and critical stage can slow down cell division and increase the risk of malformations.

In terms of development, every set of your growing baby's cells that go on to create organs and tissues are programmed to do so at a particular time during pregnancy. So if the nutrients that those specific cells need at that specific moment are lacking or insufficient, development can be compromised. Essentially, damage at this time is irreversible, so why risk it by eating in a lousy way?

Convinced? Then go back to Chapter One and take the eating plan very seriously. Your baby's future health depends on it.

Eating to beat infections

One of the many changes to occur in our bodies when pregnant is the way our immune system works. In the first sixteen weeks of pregnancy your growing baby is most vulnerable to infections that you pick up, which can be transmitted to your baby.

Given that, during pregnancy, prevention is not only better but also much less risky than a cure, it really is a good idea to try to get your immunity in great condition before and during your pregnancy.

The foods suggested in Chapter One will bolster your immunity by providing nutrients that help to fortify your external barriers to infections. In other words, they improve the strength and integrity of the linings of your nose, throat and lungs to help prevent invading bugs entering your body. They also help to shore up the strength of your internal army of infection-beating white blood cells and anti-bodies.

One other thing you can do before falling pregnant is to check on your German measles immunity. A blood test can tell if you need a quick vaccination to boost it. Go and chat with your doctor as soon as you think about falling pregnant because getting your jab three months prior to conception lowers your risk of infection once pregnant.

Eating to beat food poisoning

When it comes to food and diet, it's important to not only shore up your own resistance to infection, but also to reduce your risk of exposure to infection from bugs found in foods. This may sound odd, but the fact is, some can trigger miscarriage, stillbirth or serious health problems in a newborn baby.

Toxoplasmosis

This is caused by a parasite and is caught from eating undercooked and raw meats, unpasteurised goat's milk and cheeses, and unwashed fruits and vegetables.

This means that you must:

* **Wash your hands** before and after handling raw meat.

* **Wash** all fruits and vegetables.

* Wear **rubber gloves** if out in the garden or handling cat litter trays, since soil, mud, cats and kittens can carry this parasite.

* Only drink **heat-treated** or **pasteurised** goat's milk, yoghurt and cheeses.

Listeriosis

Listeria is a type of bacteria that can be found in **Brie**, **Camembert** and all soft cheeses with blue veins, all of which should be avoided during pregnancy and when trying to conceive. Cheddar and cottage cheese are both fine.

Paté is also off the menu, not only because it can be very high in vitamin A – which can cause birth defects – but also because it can contain listeria as well.

Ready-made salads and **ready-cooked chicken and turkey** are also all best avoided since these too can contain listeria bugs. Beware when you're eating out in chain restaurants that might buy bagged salads in bulk rather than preparing them fresh.

Ready meals are probably safe if they are kept in a properly chilled fridge and then heated up thoroughly before serving. However, if either of these elements is not watertight, listeria infection is a real possibility, so the safest option is to avoid them altogether.

Salmonella

Probably one of the better-known food poisoning bugs, the salmonella bacteria causes severe vomiting and diarrhoea that can compromise your nutrition for several days, possibly affecting your developing baby.

You can help to avoid salmonella by making sure that no raw and cooked meats or poultry touch each other during food storage and preparation. This means storing cooked meats above uncooked in the fridge, using different utensils when preparing both at the same time, and washing your hands and all surfaces when switching between the two. You also need to thoroughly cook all meat and poultry.

Chapter Three

Feeling Irie
Month One of Pregnancy

What's going on in your body?

In the seven to ten days after conception, the fertilised egg travels slowly down the Fallopian tube and attaches itself into the thickened lining of your womb (uterus). This is normally the time you would have had a period if you had not conceived, so the lack of it may be the first sign you are pregnant. What has started as a single cell (the egg) has divided time and again until it becomes a mass of 100 cells by the time it reaches your womb. It is now known as an embryo.

    Already, at this incredibly early stage, the inner part of the embryo has started growing into your baby, and the outer part is starting to develop into what will become the baby's amniotic sac and placenta. Your body will start to pump out increased levels of the female hormones oestrogen and progesterone, causing the womb lining to build up, the blood supply to the womb and breasts to increase, and the muscles of the womb to relax to make room for the growing baby. By Week Four of your pregnancy (i.e. roughly two weeks after conception), your baby is already 5 mm long and resembling a tiny tadpole, the size of a grain of rice. All this and you can't feel a thing yet!

My Diary

Lee and I lay on the bed in the small hours of the morning more awake than if we'd just knocked back triple espressos, with ridiculous Joker-like grins on our faces as our news slowly sank in. Who'd have thought, back when we first met on the BBC show (and I kissed his picture in front of my fellow judges!), that one day we'd be bringing a little person into the world together. We kept looking at each other and saying, 'Oh my God, we're going to be parents!' To think that in a couple of years' time we'd be lying in bed just as we were and a little person would come bursting through the door shouting, 'Mum, Dad!'

As the night wore on, we swapped stories about our own childhoods and what we were like when we were babies. Then I went through everything I'd been feeling over the last few weeks. The tiredness, cravings and irrationality all suddenly made sense. There was one particular situation where I'd behaved completely out of character that I was now able to explain. Having opened in many theatre shows I'm used to receiving both good and bad reviews – it's the nature of the business – but the show I was doing in Edinburgh had received bad press from a couple of female journalists, one of whom I happened to recognise. The morning after the show opened I was having breakfast with friends in a coffee shop when in walked this particular journalist. My mates literally had to hold me back to stop me from going over to confront her and give her a face full of Eggs Benedict. It was totally unlike me but I could now put it down to the raging hormones.

Lee and I continued excitedly jabbering away about the future into the night without an ounce of anxiety or apprehension, just pure joy mixed with a gradual realisation that our lives were going to change drastically. After all, I'd spent the last thirty-five years only having to worry about myself, getting up when I liked and jetting off when I fancied a quick break. In fact the very next day I was off for a girly pampering trip with my dear friend Lucy, to the sunny Caribbean island of Jamaica. We'd been planning the trip for ages and I needed the holiday so much after my stint in Edinburgh. To say I'd been looking forward to it was an understatement, but it felt weird to be leaving Lee so soon after we'd discovered our happy news. Saying goodbye to him was hard but, as he pointed out, he had a manic week of work ahead so it would be best for me to get away and relax in the sunshine.

Needless to say, I was up super-bright and early the following morning with a spring in my step. Before I left for the airport, I called my doctors to tell them I was pregnant and that I was due to go on holiday in a couple of hours. They told me not to worry, to enjoy my time away, and they booked me an appointment for a week's time.

After years of friendship, Lucy knows me well enough to tell when I'm hiding something, and it didn't take long for me to crack after I arrived at the airport. Perhaps my huge grin had something to do with giving it away. We found somewhere quiet and I told her our fantastic news. She was overjoyed and was equally happy that our planned cocktail-fuelled week would now be one of relaxation, healthy eating and baby talk.

Taking care not to be caught out by inquisitive shoppers and to risk any premature phone calls to the press, we went all *A-Team* and Lucy did all my shopping for preggy mags and books in the airport, surreptitiously slipping them to me on board when the coast was clear. With the magazines came the sudden realisation that there is so much to do and so many things to consider, and my baby-carrying bliss soon turned into minor panic as all the kids on board started screaming in unison, like some kind of manic chorus line sent to warn me of what lay ahead. As I noticed the tired faces of stressed-out mums throughout the plane I had my first 'Are we really ready for this?' moment.

A couple of hours at the villa and the relaxation kicked in ('Club Tropicana' on the iPod certainly helped). Our villa was really tranquil and had its own lovely pool for Lucy and I to chill in. Each morning I'd wake up early and lie there for a moment before it dawned on me that I was pregnant. It was a great feeling, like finding out all over again. It's always easier to eat more healthily when you're in a lovely warm climate with plenty of delicious fresh fruit available, but from day one I was absolutely focused on maintaining a healthy diet for the baby. Oh my gosh – the baby! It still seemed so surreal.

Every day started with a healthy breakfast of fruit and cereal before heading to the pool for a dip and gentle swim. The sun was so strong that I'd only sit in it for a few minutes during the early morning, feeling my stomach gently warming up, before heading to the shade. There I'd lie, blissfully flicking through all the pregnancy magazines, devouring every piece of advice – learning what I needed to do, the best things to eat and what was to come. I felt like I'd just received membership for an exciting new club.

Lunchtimes and dinners soon had their own little routine too. I'd carefully explain at each restaurant that I was pregnant and the waiters would help me out with pregnancy-friendly alternatives to the menu where necessary. Between the staff, my newfound knowledge from the magazines and the ever-helpful Google on my Blackberry, there was very little chance of me going anywhere near food that wasn't super-healthy for both me and the baby, and I was certainly in the right place for good-quality food. Every day I'd opt for fresh fruit and vegetables and locally caught fish, and I quickly became addicted to a huge salad, which was full of everything from cheese and avocado to incredibly juicy fruit. My appetite had gone through the roof so not only was I tucking away my own meals but I'd also help Lucy out with hers – but hey, that's what friends are for. What I couldn't work out was why all the magazines were saying I shouldn't be 'eating for two'. I was starving! Maybe it's a psychological thing: us girls are normally so worried about how much we eat that as soon as we have an excuse to let go a bit we grab it with both hands.

My biggest problem at this point was forcing myself to stay properly hydrated without spending all day on the loo. Let's be honest, who's a big fan of drinking several litres of water every day? I've certainly never enjoyed it but now I didn't have a choice, so it was a case of squeezing fresh Jamaican lemons and limes into ice-cold water. I have to admit that even I found that quite refreshing.

It wasn't until we were halfway through our week that it dawned on me: I hadn't yet experienced the slightest bit of morning sickness. Why it's called morning sickness baffles me anyway, as some of my mates had it morning, noon and night throughout their pregnancies and for the whole nine months. The only times I'd felt slightly nauseous so far were if I hadn't eaten for a couple of hours and my stomach felt empty. Maybe I had it to come, who knows? After all, this was only just the start of a really exciting journey and I was prepared to embrace it all. Part of me wanted to experience it, almost as a validation of my being pregnant, but at the same time growing a baby without any accompanying morning sickness seemed like a lovely ideal.

Early evenings spent sitting outside the villa were just magical, as the most stunning sunset would light up the sky over the Caribbean Sea. I'd sit there drinking coconut water, missing Lee but content in the knowledge that our family was expanding and we had a lifetime of fun and adventures to come. I'd call Lee every day to let him know I was OK and we'd chat away for ages. It was lovely to hear his excitement and I felt reassured that he was getting emotionally involved so early on. He was going to make a great dad.

Towards the end of the week, just in case there was so much as an ounce of stress that had managed to elude my attempts to reach new heights of relaxation, I booked myself a massage. I explained to the therapist that I was pregnant and that she should take extra care around my belly. It seemed very strange that in the early stages of pregnancy you end up telling complete strangers about this amazing news and yet family and close friends were yet to find out, but sometimes it's unavoidable. I just couldn't wait to share our secret with our nearest and dearest.

Our wonderful week in paradise flew past, but by the time our last day arrived I wasn't just feeling relaxed but also very excited about getting home. As beautiful as Jamaica was, I couldn't wait to get back to see Lee, visit my doctor and find out just how many weeks' pregnant I was.

Now for the Experts...

Exercising in the first trimester (weeks one to thirteen)

If you're new to exercise, start with twenty minutes of brisk walking every day, or half an hour three times a week. Alternatively you could swim for twenty minutes, two or three times a week. Otherwise, continue with your normal exercise programme, as outlined in the previous chapter.

Don't feel that you have to give up weight lifting, aerobics or even spinning if you are pregnant. Just use your common sense as to which sports you can continue with (see the Don'ts list below for pointers). In general, keeping your regular fitness routine intact is the best thing you can do for you and your baby, though of course you will need to modify your regime to keep it at a mild to moderate level. If you become tired or uncomfortable doing your normal activities, switch to something gentle such as stretching or yoga.

However, do bear in mind that even if you were in great shape before you got pregnant, there are occasions when exercise during pregnancy may be strictly forbidden to protect your health, your baby's health, or both. If you have any of the following conditions either now or later on in the pregnancy, consult a doctor. You'll probably be advised not to exercise while pregnant.

- **Pregnancy-induced hypertension** (high blood pressure)
- **Pre-term rupture of membranes**
- **Pre-term labour,** now or during a prior pregnancy
- **Incompetent cervix**
- **Persistent second or third trimester bleeding**
- **Intrauterine growth retardation**
- **Heart disease**

Exercising when newly pregnant – dos and don'ts

DO:

✽ **Check** with your GP or midwife before you start exercising.

✽ Keep your **fluid levels** up so you don't dehydrate.

✽ Wear loose, comfortable **clothing** and a supportive bra, and make sure you don't overheat.

✽ Watch your **posture** and use your tummy muscles to support your back while exercising.

✽ **Keep moving**: avoid doing anything that involves standing motionless for long periods as it can decrease blood flow to the uterus. If you are doing something fairly static such as weight lifting, change positions regularly.

✽ Seek out **antenatal exercise** programmes where the instructors are specifically trained to help you and there are other pregnant women in the class for support and inspiration.

✽ Make sure you can carry on a **conversation** while exercising. This is called the 'talk test'. You have less oxygen available for aerobic exercise when you're pregnant, so slow down if you can't talk comfortably.

✽ Monitor your **heart rate**. During pregnancy, it should not exceed 140 beats per minute or sixty per cent of your maximum heart rate. Your heart beats faster during pregnancy, so bear in mind you won't have to exercise as hard to reach your target rate.

❊ Take lots of time to **relax** and breathe deeply after you've exercised. Deep 'belly breathing' will help you during childbirth as well as helping you to feel calm.

DON'T:

❊ Don't exercise to **extremes**. In any case, research shows that little and often gives better results than harder, less frequent exercise.

❊ Don't do any exercise while pregnant that could result in **abdominal trauma**. So waterskiing, snowboarding, horse-riding and contact sports are out, and be wary of continuing with cycling or jogging on uneven surfaces. Instead, exercise in safe environments where you can control what goes on.

❊ If you've been training for a **sports event** before you were pregnant, switch the focus to training for you and your baby rather than on the event itself. There's no need to abandon your goal completely (unless it's potentially dangerous or highly competitive) but you will need to take it more easily.

❊ Don't do **ab crunches**. These can cause excessive strain to your torso and could actually make your abs *less* flat after birth!

❊ Don't **scuba dive** or go to high altitudes. (Do we really need to tell you this?!)

❋ Don't exercise for long periods in the **supine position** (lying flat on your back) after the first trimester. This position decreases blood flow to the uterus. Rest for forty to sixty seconds and then move.

❋ Don't continue to exercise if you have any of the **following symptoms**: dizziness or fainting, shortness of breath, vaginal bleeding, sudden water discharge, signs of labour, headaches, chest pain, calf pain or swelling, rapid heartbeat while resting. Stop immediately and seek medical assistance. Later in your pregnancy you will also need to be aware of your baby's movements in the womb – if there is an unusual absence of foetal movements, stop exercising (though bear in mind that the baby is most often quiet when you are on the move).

❋ Similarly, don't exercise if you feel any **pain**. Stop immediately, and if the pain persists, seek professional help.

❋ Don't **over-stretch** or push too hard. When you are pregnant, your joints are less stable and more vulnerable to sprains due to the pregnancy hormone *relaxin*, which loosens all the ligaments and pelvic joints in preparation for childbirth. For the same reason, avoid sports that might throw you off-balance.

❋ Don't have a **sauna**, or go in a hot tub or steam room. All have the potential to raise your core body temperature, which, early in pregnancy, has been associated with foetal neural tube defects like spina bifida. Hyperthermia (temperature greater than 102 degrees Fahrenheit) has also been associated with miscarriage, foetal growth restriction and brain damage.

Pelvic floor exercises

If there's one thing you should do throughout your pregnancy it's pelvic floor exercises! These help you to avoid stress incontinence (leaking urine) during pregnancy and, after the baby is born, reduce the risk of vaginal prolapse. They also improve blood circulation to the genital area, which improves sexual arousal. You will want sex again one day. Honestly.

To find your pelvic floor, sit on the loo, clench the muscles that stop you weeing, and release them. These are your PC muscles. Now imagine a zip inside your lower abdomen, or an elevator going up a lift shaft and stopping at three different floors. Contract the muscles, hold for four to five seconds, squeeze the lift up to the next floor, hold for four to five seconds, then squeeze again, holding once more. When you reach the top, don't just let go of the muscles. Instead, start descending to each floor, again holding for four to five seconds at each stage.

Try to do this at least five times a day; ten after you've had the baby. If you're prone to forgetting, do them whenever you stop at a red light, bus stop or train station.

Pregnancy massages

As Denise found in Jamaica, a pregnancy massage can decrease stress and improve relaxation, aid lymph drainage, and have a balancing effect on glands, all of which are of huge benefit during pregnancy. Furthermore, massages can release endorphins, promote muscle elasticity, reduce fatigue, minimise spider veins and even alleviate symptoms of morning sickness, and it is believed they help your body to eliminate harmful toxins and allow your cells to maximise the absorption of valuable nutrients. It's no surprise, therefore, that massage can be an important tool in a healthy and happy pregnancy.

However, as beneficial as a maternity massage can be, it is critical that your massage is carried out by a properly qualified therapist, who is trained to work on pregnant women. A badly executed massage can put you at risk of miscarriage.

The myth of 'eating for two'

It is true, unfortunately: after all those years of old wives, mothers and grandmothers telling us that we should be 'eating for two', that particular excuse to 'go for it' with cream cakes and chocolate Hob Nobs has now been exposed for the **myth** it is.

The truth is, if you are a normal weight when you begin your pregnancy, you only actually need an additional **200–300 calories** a day in the last three months.

While this may be a bit of shock, it begins to make sense when you look at the maths. On the one hand your basic speed of metabolism (and therefore the amount of calories you burn each day) increases slightly when you're pregnant, because your body is busy making the placenta, building up extra fat supplies and, of course, making your baby. You also burn more calories getting around because there is more of you, just as a big Bentley uses more fuel than a small Smart car.

On the other hand, this increased need for calories is made up for by the fact that you tend to actually move less in pregnancy than in your normal day-to-day life. In addition, your normal post-meal 'jump' in metabolism is slightly reduced, which 'saves' calories.

The combined effect of decreased movement and metabolic changes during pregnancy helps to ensure that we can sustain a foetus if food is not in good supply. In other words, these are brilliant adaptations to ensure that our pregnancy can proceed even under difficult nutritional circumstances.

The problem is that here in the West many of us have access to *too much* food, rather than not enough, so we need to be aware that pregnancy is not a time to abuse our bodies by going crazy and overfilling it with calories it simply does not need.

There are two particularly good reasons for not pigging out on junk. **Firstly** you are less likely to be left with the Herculean task of trying to lose loads of weight post-birth. **Secondly** and most importantly, poor nutrition can potentially have a negative effect on your baby's future health, both immediately and as he grows up and moves into adulthood.

We know from studies on pregnant women that the more weight that the mother puts on in pregnancy, the higher the risk that her child will grow up to be obese. There is also some fascinating research, albeit in animals, that shows that mothers who eat an unhealthy diet while pregnant may be putting their offspring at risk of developing long-term (but not irreversible) health problems, including type 2 diabetes, raised cholesterol, high blood sugar and obesity. Rodents that were fed a diet rich in fat, sugar and salt while pregnant were more likely to give birth to offspring that over-ate and had a preference for junk food when compared to the offspring of rats given regular food. It seems that a mother's diet may have a lasting effect on her child's body, causing it to metabolise food differently (even when weaned off junk food) well beyond adolescence.

We all know the saying 'you are what you eat'; well, this research suggests that it may be that 'you are what your mother ate'. If this research turns out to be true for humans too – and there is no reason why it should not, given that we share a number of fundamental biological systems with rats – then there is no better reason for eating well during pregnancy and not giving in to cravings for junk or eating for two.

How much weight should I gain when pregnant?

This is a difficult question to answer. If you are a normal weight when you fall pregnant, the British Dietetic Association recommends that you should gain at least **10–12 kg** (1 stone 8 lb to 1 stone 12 lb). If you are overweight, then **6.8 kg** (1 stone 1 lb) should be enough.

You should not try to lose weight during pregnancy, whatever your starting weight, because doing so may affect the mental development of your baby, especially in the second half of pregnancy.

Where does the extra weight go?

According to the Royal College of Obstetrics and Gynaecologists, the following gains occur in our bodies when pregnant (though bear in mind these figures can vary widely depending on your genetics, starting weight and so on):

Uterus	**0.9 kg** (2 lb approx)
Breasts	**0.4 kg** (1 lb approx)
Blood	**1.2 kg** (2½ lb approx)
Extracellular fluid	**1.2 kg** (2½ lb approx)
Fat	**3.5 kg** (7½ lb approx)

Your baby will add around another 3.6 kg (8 lb) by full term.

Morning Sickness

Denise was one of the lucky ones not to experience morning sickness. Nausea and vomiting affect around fifty per cent of pregnant women, beginning as early on as four weeks into the pregnancy, although it tends to be more often around weeks six to eight. It tends to peak between weeks eight to twelve, and then wears off.

Morning sickness can put you off your food, which means that you have to make a really big effort to ensure that you do still take in as much of a healthy diet as possible, even though you may not feel like eating. If you are vomiting, be particularly careful: your growing baby needs vital nutrients to develop optimally, which can be lost through vomiting.

Unfortunately there is no really good, fail-safe advice on dealing with morning sickness, but there are some things which may help to alleviate symptoms:

✤ Having an empty stomach makes it worse, so eating **dry snacks** every couple of hours may help. Try some toast with sugar-free jam but no butter, plain biscuits like Rich Tea and oatcakes, a baked potato with no filling, or low-fat fromage frais and fruit salads.

✤ Keep your rooms **well ventilated** both at home and at work, and don't get out of bed too quickly in the morning.

✤ **Ginger** is well known by medical herbalists to help in the treatment of nausea. It appears to boost digestive juices and neutralise acids, which helps alleviate symptoms. But be careful how much you take in: a few ginger biscuits or a cup of ginger tea daily is OK in the first two months of pregnancy, but you shouldn't try more than this unless you seek the advice of your GP first.

✤ Finally, morning sickness provides another good reason to take a daily **multivitamin and mineral supplement** designed for pregnancy, to ensure that at least your basic nutritional needs are still being met. If you suffer from very bad morning sickness, do speak to your GP.

Chapter Four

Secrets and Lies
Month Two of Pregnancy

What's going on in your body?

By Week Five of your pregnancy, your baby's nervous system is starting to develop, the heart is forming, and blood vessels are sprouting, creating the beginnings of an umbilical cord connecting the placenta to the baby. By Week Seven the baby will be the size of a baked bean: about 10 mm long from head to bottom. The first signs of ears and eyes appear on the embryo, and little bumps are forming where the arms and legs will grow. The heart begins to beat and can be seen on an ultrasound.

As for you, you may get some light 'spotting' at this stage (a small amount of blood) but this is a normal side effect of the embryo implanting into your womb, so nothing to worry about as long as it stops after a day or so. You may also have sore boobs, some nausea or vomiting, extreme tiredness, a sudden sensitivity to your normal food, drink or smells, or the need to wee more often than usual. Get used to it – you'll be feeling a lot more of these things over the coming months...

My Diary

My stay in Jamaica was amazing and much needed, but arriving home again at such a special time felt fantastic. There was nowhere else I would rather have been at that point than in what was soon to become our family home.

A trip to see Dr Silverstone confirmed that I was indeed eight weeks' pregnant. My very first scan was amazing. I rolled down my jeggings to expose my tanned tummy, prompting the sonographer Dr Pran to ask me if I had had a nice holiday. He then squeezed cold gel on to my tummy and smeared it around with a funny-shaped object that I now know to be a transducer, which sends and receives the ultrasound waves (listen to me, getting all technical). A bit of manoeuvring and there was our little kidney bean of a baby on the screen, its tiny heart racing away. I couldn't help but shed a tear or ten and Lee was beaming with pride, which made me cry even more. Thank the Lord for waterproof mascara. Despite the middle-of-the-night pee-stick drama, the last week of excitement and a mountain of baby magazines, only now did it start to feel very real.

We floated out of the surgery with huge smiles across our faces, happy in the knowledge that everything was healthy, I was definitely pregnant, the pregnancy test hadn't been a dud and I hadn't just reached an age when my weight was starting to balloon.

It was action stations straight away as we headed to the chemist to pick up some folic acid on doctor's orders and, continuing with the healthy eating trend, we also had a major stock-up on fresh fruit and veg. I'd never been so excited about buying broccoli and carrots in my life – the poor greengrocer must have thought I was bonkers as I dashed around the shop squeezing and examining his wares to make sure everything was super-fresh, letting out sporadic bursts of song as I went. Now I was part of the mum-to-be club it seemed a necessity. I was determined to do everything I could to stay as healthy as possible to give our baby the best start in life.

That evening, over a meal of fresh fish and vegetables, Lee and I discussed when would be the best time to tell our families and close friends. I was dying to shout our news from the rooftops there and then but, taking on board the advice from the magazines I'd read and remembering what other pregnant friends had done, we agreed it was best to hold fire. Like many couples in this situation, we decided that we should wait until after I'd reached the twelve-week point to announce it to the world, when the risk of a miscarriage is greatly reduced. That seemed like the sensible thing to do, especially as my sister had experienced difficulties during a pregnancy in the past and it could be something that ran in the family. That said, we wanted to tell our immediate families straight away as we felt it would be important to have their advice and support. I called my mum and dad first and they were thrilled for us – though they already have four grandchildren so were a bit matter-of-fact once the news had sunk in. I think they were also half-expecting my call as they knew we were trying. It was only a few weeks earlier that my brother and sister-in-law had announced they were expecting and my mum mentioned that she had seen the brief flicker of disappointment in my face before I broke into a smile. Obviously I was delighted for them but at the same time I was wondering when it would be our turn.

The Meads were *super*-excited. Lee is one of two boys and his brother Casey is yet to start a family, so Lee's parents were keen to begin spreading the news of their first grandchild straight away. We explained to them that we wanted to wait another month before telling anyone outside of the immediate family and they agreed – mum would be the word.

I also told a couple of my closest friends so I could turn to them for advice if I needed it. I heard so many different pregnancy stories – I had one friend, who shall remain nameless to protect her identity, who showed me first-hand the full force of morning sickness. I'd been waiting for her in our favourite restaurant, salivating over everything on the menu. When she turned up I'd just stood up to give her a hug when her face suddenly changed, and with a look of panic she turned and ran out of the restaurant. I dashed out behind her to find her at the side of the kerb, bent over and retching. As I leant down beside her, holding her hair, we must have looked like a couple of girls who'd started early on the booze.

One of the close friends I confided in, my mate Karen, was due to give birth the following month to a baby girl so she was delighted we were going to experience the journey of motherhood together. It was Karen who had very kindly passed the 'magic book' on to me a few months earlier, which I had forgotten about completely. Before falling pregnant she had been trying to conceive for two years, and was getting desperate until a friend gave her a huge book on the technicalities of pregnancy. Apparently it was 'magic' and every girl to take the book into her home had subsequently fallen pregnant. I was the eighth girl to become pregnant after receiving the book and – call me superstitious – I have since passed it on to my friend Sam and she's proudly sporting a bump right now. Don't get me wrong, you don't need to *read* the book (which is just as well, as it looked more like instructions to fly to the moon than advice on the best way to conceive) – just having it in the house seems to work.

With our families and a few close friends in on our secret we now had four weeks to keep it from anyone else. Goodness knows how that was supposed to happen, as I'm officially the worst person in the world when it comes to accidentally letting secrets slip. I actually found it hardest to keep it from my work colleagues. My diary was busier than ever and I was having to make up excuse after excuse for everything from my weight gain and constant trips to the loo, to my general ditziness (although some may say I've always lived up to the reputation blondes have).

One of my jobs where I had to be creative with the truth (sounds much better than 'tell lies') was a presenting job for Channel Four. I'm a massive fan of Kylie so of course I jumped at the chance to host an hour-long documentary celebrating her life. But first I needed a suitable outfit to wear, something in keeping with Kylie's young and funky style. I visited one of my favourite stores, but as the assistant pulled out loads of lycra in a size small/medium I just froze. Once in the safety of the changing room I decided I might as well try on some of the clothes she'd selected for me. Big mistake – just one leg squeezed into a pair of super-tight PVC leggings confirmed that I had more chance of becoming the next Kylie myself than getting my other leg, not to mention my bum, into any of the outfits. Despite my panic I still managed to muster a laugh and a reassuring rub on my belly as I peeled my leg out of the lycra before the lack of blood circulation did any serious damage.

It was no good. I had to say something. I peered around the curtain to see the young girl's expectant face looking back at me, no doubt waiting for me to bound out of the changing room declaring how much I loved the selection of clothes. I took a deep breath before saying the phrase we women dread having to say: 'Can I try all of these in a larger size please?' The assistant looked at me with a slight hesitation as if she were about to try and persuade me I didn't need to go up a size, before nodding her head and dashing off back into the shop. Phew, she'd got the message, even if it had felt like I had just been to confession ('Forgive me, shop assistant, for I have sinned: my bum and thighs have grown').

Filming the documentary wasn't any easier thanks to what I soon found out was endearingly known as 'baby brain'. I'd heard pregnant friends mention their forgetfulness in the past but I hadn't realised just how bad it could be. Only a matter of weeks ago I was staging an hour-long one-woman show with ease, yet right now I was finding it almost impossible to learn a few lines of my script. One moment they'd be in my head, then in the time it would take for the director to call 'Action!', they'd vanish. Unfortunately we were filming in various locations around London so I didn't have an autocue, that oh-so-handy device on the camera that displays your lines. I was tripping over my words and getting all the names of Kylie's songs wrong. Have you heard 'Love At Sirst Fight'? Or indulged in the 'Local-potion' on the dancefloor?

By the time we got to early afternoon I was exhausted, the outfit I had miraculously squeezed into felt like it was getting tighter by the minute, and my feet were throbbing. I just wanted to curl up in a ball and fall asleep in a corner somewhere. But I had managed to get through the day, and my reward when I got home was a warm bubble bath and a super-early night.

The next big hurdle for me to blag my way through was a team photoshoot for a 1,000-mile cycle ride in aid of Sport Relief. Before I'd found out I was pregnant I'd signed up to participate in the bike ride alongside two of my close friends, Fearne Cotton and David Walliams. How could I have said no, it was for such a great cause and would no doubt be a real hoot. Of course cycling so far while pregnant wouldn't be wise, so I would have to drop out before the actual event, but if I hadn't turned up for the initial shoot I would have had to face a barrage of questions from organisers and the press. As a result, it was best foot forward for this one.

When I arrived at the shoot the coordinator explained that they wanted me to get on a pogo stick and jump around. A pogo stick – you have *got* to be kidding me! Now I'm no obstetrician but I'm pretty sure that, in the early stages of pregnancy, bouncing up and down repeatedly would be considered unwise. Of course I wasn't going to take that kind of risk so my ongoing back trouble (from which I genuinely do suffer) became my excuse. In the end they settled for the slightly more sedate version of me running with a little jump in the air, though even then I was still worried I was doing something I shouldn't be.

I was also asked to revisit Uganda to see first-hand the benefits brought from the money we had raised from climbing Mount Kilimanjaro. I would have absolutely loved to have gone on the trip but the list of vaccinations was pretty scary even if you're not pregnant so that was just something else I had to talk my way round. I guess telling the organisers that I had signed up to play a mum in a new soap wasn't too far from the truth.

I was becoming a pro at 'misleading' people in my work and social life and wasn't enjoying it in the slightest. Both Lee and I were telling so many white lies it was getting confusing. I was on antibiotics; I was the designated driver for the evening; I had a super-early start – these were just a few of my stock excuses for not having a glass of wine with friends. Cancelling nights out and avoiding phone calls also became regular practice during that period. It may only have been four weeks but it seemed like an eternity. I was so relieved when we reached the final week of having to keep our wonderful secret but I have to admit to feeling slightly worried about how people would now treat me once the word got out. Showbiz can be a fickle industry.

Now for the Experts...

As Denise found, belly expansion is inevitable in pregnancy. Around the third month of pregnancy, most women will find that their clothes will become tight around the waist. You will generally need to be wearing maternity clothing by the fourth or fifth month.

Of course, some people are less fortunate than others and find that their belly expands very rapidly when pregnant. This might be because they were overweight before pregnancy (or conversely that they were very slender beforehand, which makes the bump 'show' more); they are carrying multiple babies; it's their second or subsequent pregnancy; they are bloated (often caused by not drinking enough water); or simply that they are eating too much and therefore gaining weight too quickly. Rarely, rapid belly expansion can be a sign of an underlying health issue such as a liver problem or a cyst, so check with your doctor if you're concerned. Just remember that everyone's bump is different so there's no point comparing yourself to other pregnant women (indeed your own bump may look completely different in any subsequent pregnancies).

Some common problems caused by rapid belly expansion:

✳ **Stretch marks.** The faster your tum expands, the more likely you are to get stretch marks. Stretch marks can be itchy and unsightly, but if you're troubled by them you can ask your doctor who may be able to recommend a safe stretch mark cream for you.

✳ **Negative body image.** Let's face it, no one wants to 'balloon' suddenly, particularly if you haven't yet told people that you're expecting. Feeling fat and frumpy when pregnant is perfectly normal, but depressing nonetheless. Invest some time and money tracking down flattering maternity clothes – they will do wonders for your self-esteem.

❊ **Shortness of breath and backaches.** This is very common in pregnancy: see below for some ideas to help.

Pregnancy back pain

Denise has always suffered with back problems. But even if you've never had back pain before (and you're not being asked to jump around on a pogo stick), unfortunately almost all pregnant women at one point or another will suffer from this unpleasant problem.

Backache in early pregnancy is caused by the extra weight you are carrying and your new lower centre of gravity, both of which conspire to put added pressure on your back. It's also an unfortunate side effect of the pregnancy hormone relaxin, which loosens up the ligaments around your pelvis. While this is helpful for allowing your uterus to expand as the baby grows, the increased flexibility does leave you vulnerable to back pain from strains and injuries. Your abdominal wall also changes as your baby grows: it stretches and becomes thinner, and your abdominal muscles – that normally help to stabilise the back – grow weaker.

Sometimes you will feel shooting pains in your lower back and legs. This is due to *sciatica*, which is when the baby's head presses down on the sciatic nerve (the body's longest nerve, that runs from the backbone through the pelvis and down towards the leg). If you've ever suffered from this, you will know it is agony.

So, what can be done? Toning and strengthening the back and abdominal muscles through a stretching routine and moderate exercise programme can usually help. A stretching routine is also very good for toning the perineal area, stretching ligaments, strengthening the inner thigh and abdominal muscles and promoting proper body alignment, all of which will help keep lower-back pain and sciatica at bay. If you are already suffering, try the following self-help measures or the stretches listed below.

* **Get moving**. As outlined above, any activity that gently strengthens and stretches the muscles in your back and legs will help, especially in early pregnancy.

* **Sit up straight** and avoid slouching. Try to take regular breaks to move around which will help stretch your muscles. Sit with your feet slightly raised on a footstool whenever possible.

* Try sitting on a **fitness ball** if you need to sit at a desk for a long period of time. You may get some funny looks, but these spacehopper-like balls are excellent at helping you to position your body properly, and they can reduce backache.

* Always **bend** from the knees when you lift anything, and try to avoid lifting anything heavy.

* Use extra **pillows** when resting or sleeping to support your body – try lying on your side with a pillow propped between your legs.

* Soak in a **warm bath** to relieve aches and pains (though not too hot – and avoid hot tubs while pregnant). Hot and cold packs applied directly to your aches and pains can help relax strained muscles and ligaments.

* Ditch the **high heels** for the time being (sorry, girls).

Stretches for the lower back

Squatting Stretch

This is a great stretch and toner for
your legs and perineal muscles.

1 Stand against a table or other
   piece of furniture.

2 Using one hand to support
   yourself, squat down slowly for
   one minute at a time, ten times
   a day.

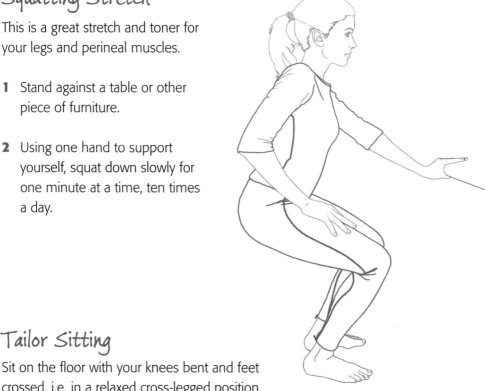

Tailor Sitting

Sit on the floor with your knees bent and feet
crossed, i.e. in a relaxed cross-legged position.
Spend ten minutes at least two or three times a
day sitting in this position. It will stretch your inner thighs and takes the
pressure off your lower back. A variation of this is to sit on the floor with
your knees bent and your back supported against the sofa or a wall. Put
your feet together, sole to sole. Slowly, move your knees down and see
how close to the floor you can get them.

The Pelvic Tilt

This stretch gives relief from lower-back pain and also helps prepare the body for birth.

1   Lie on your back with your knees bent and feet flat on the floor.

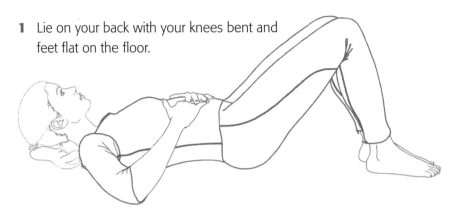

2   Exhale while pressing the small of your back against the floor then inhale and relax the spine. Repeat this several times.

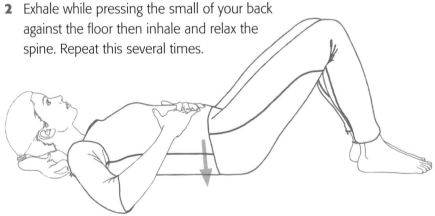

After the fourth month of pregnancy, do this stretch in a standing position against the wall, by pressing the small of the back against the wall and then relaxing. This avoids you having to lie on your back, which is not recommended in later pregnancy.

Arched Cat

This stretch relieves the pressure of the enlarged uterus on the spine.

1 Get down on your hands and knees on the floor.

2 Keeping your head straight and
neck relaxed and aligned
with the spine, arch the back
upwards like a cat while
tightening the abdomen and
buttocks inwards. Allow your
head to drop
down.

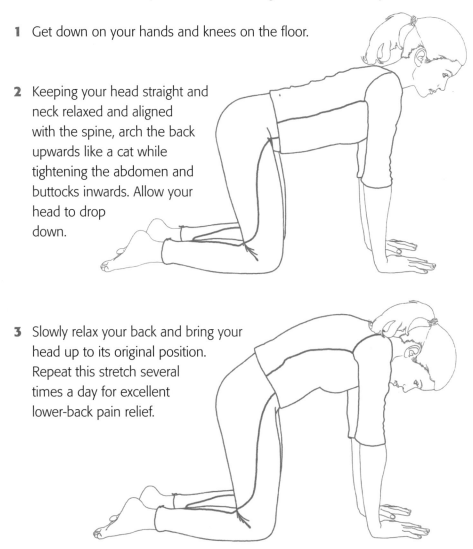

3 Slowly relax your back and bring your
head up to its original position.
Repeat this stretch several
times a day for excellent
lower-back pain relief.

Foods to avoid while pregnant

It's difficult to say 'no' to foods when you are pregnant, especially when not everyone knows your secret yet, as Denise found. But unfortunately, certain foods can put your health or your baby's at risk, so you need to avoid them both while trying to become pregnant and once you actually are.

Never feel as though you are being a 'nuisance' when declining foods and drinks. It is your baby's health at stake. If you upset someone in the process, whether it is a relative, friend or member of staff in a restaurant, then so be it. They will get over it. Your baby may not.

So here is the list. It may seem a bit overwhelming at first but don't worry. Try jotting this list down in a notebook or diary so that you can refer to it when you're out and about.

Fish

Shark, **swordfish** and **marlin** are completely off the menu while pregnant. This is because these large fish are pretty much at the top of the marine food chain and have had a lot of time during their lives to collect quite high levels of methyl mercury in their flesh. If you eat these fish then your mercury levels can rise, which can be passed on through your placenta to your growing baby, and in turn affect its developing nervous system.

Tuna is another large fish, so again you need to watch for mercury levels. It doesn't pose quite so much of a threat, so you can eat a limited amount: up to two tuna steaks a week (170 g uncooked weight and 140 g cooked weight), or up to four medium-sized cans of tuna a week (140 g drained weight).

Oily fish – including salmon, mackerel, sardines, pilchards, anchovies, trout and fresh (not canned) tuna – can harbour environmental pollutants called dioxins and PCBs in their fat stores, which are distributed throughout their flesh. Dioxins and PCBs can also be found in sea bream, sea bass, turbot, halibut, huss (also known as rock salmon, flake, rock eel or dogfish), as well as brown crabmeat. These pollutants can build up in our fat cells and pass across the placenta when we consume them, which may disrupt the delicate development of organs and tissues and the hormone levels in our growing baby.

You may feel safer just to avoid all fish having read this, but that would be a shame because things like cod and plaice and well-cooked shellfish like prawns are great sources of protein and are low in fat. They also give us important minerals like iodine, which is needed for the healthy growth of your baby. In addition, having a portion of oily fish once a week will help to provide you with omega 3 essential fats that are crucial for the development of your baby's eyes, hearing and brain.

If you want to avoid all oily fish, then ask your GP or health visitor about the benefits of taking an omega 3 supplement so that you do not lose out on these vital fats. You need to find one that is as free as possible of pollutants or one that is based on marine algae.

Flax seed does provide omega 3s, but they are not well utilised by our bodies.

Cheese

As mentioned in Chapter Two, **Brie**, **Camembert**, **chèvre** (goats' cheese) and other cheeses that have a thick white rind should be avoided, along with cheeses with blue veins. This is because they can contain the bacteria called listeria, which can be damaging to your unborn baby.

The good news is that feta, Cheddar, mozzarella, cottage and ricotta cheeses, cheese spreads, cream cheese and mascarpone are all fine, although it is worth going steady on serving sizes so that you do not overdo total saturated fat intakes and calories.

Patés and liver

Patés should be avoided because they too can contain listeria. Also, if they are made from liver, they are very likely to be high in vitamin A, which can cause birth defects in your developing baby.

Raw eggs, meat and shellfish

Raw eggs (e.g. in home-made mayonnaise) and undercooked eggs should be avoided because they can contain salmonella. This can cause vomiting and diarrhoea, which, while not directly harmful to your baby, are unpleasant for you and can put you off your food, reducing nutrient supply to your growing baby. Ditto **raw shellfish** and **raw or undercooked meat** – so make sure you avoid things like steak tartare and check that burgers, chicken and so on are well cooked all the way through to avoid food poisoning.

Caffeine

You should limit yourself to no more than **200 mg of caffeine** per day. As a rule, you find 100 mg of caffeine in a cup of coffee and up to 150 mg in a mug. A cup of tea has around 75 mg and a large mug has up to 100 mg.

But it's not just tea and coffee that contain caffeine. Cans of **cola** have around 40 mg of caffeine each, while a 250 ml can of energy drink can have more than double or even triple this amount. A 50 g bar of **dark chocolate** contains around 40 mg of caffeine while the same portion of milk chocolate has about 20 mg. **Coffee-flavour ice creams** can also contain caffeine, as can **cold remedies**, so always check the labels.

Peanuts

These only need to be avoided if you have a peanut allergy yourself. The official advice on this has changed quite a bit over the years, but this is the current recommendation that came into being in August 2009.

Honey

This is fine for pregnant women; though babies under one year of age should avoid it because it can contain a type of bacterial spore capable of producing toxins that can lead to infant botulism and serious illness.

The low-down on alcohol

Denise was wise to avoid alcohol during her pregnancy. It is a bit of a hot potato as to whether the 'odd' single unit of alcohol is OK occasionally, or if we should abstain totally. Perhaps the best thing is to reproduce what the various health bodies say on the subject both here and in America, then you can decide on the best course of action for you. (One unit, incidentally, is half a pint of standard strength beer, lager or cider, or a pub measure of spirit. A 175 ml glass of 12% wine is about two units and alcopops are about one and a half units.)

British Dietetic Association: 'It is unknown what levels of alcohol are safe in pregnancy. Alcohol is best avoided throughout pregnancy and especially if planning a pregnancy and during the first three months. If you do choose to have alcohol, limit it to one or two units once or twice a week and avoid getting drunk or binge drinking (over five units).'

Royal College of Obstetrics and Gynaecologists in the UK:
'When a woman drinks during her pregnancy, the alcohol passes from her bloodstream through the placenta and into the baby's bloodstream. The safest approach in pregnancy is not to drink at all. Small amounts of alcohol during pregnancy (not more than one to two units, not more than once to twice a week) have not shown to be harmful. Regular binge drinking around conception and in early pregnancy is particularly harmful to a woman and her baby.'

The American College of Obstetrics and Gynaecology:
'ACOG reiterates its long-standing position that no amount of alcohol consumption can be considered safe during pregnancy. Women should avoid alcohol entirely while pregnant or trying to conceive because damage can occur in the earliest weeks of pregnancy, even before a woman knows that she is pregnant.'

The American Dietetic Association: 'Alcohol should not be consumed by pregnant women or by those who may become pregnant. Drinking during pregnancy is associated with major neurological and developmental birth defects. Even moderate drinking during pregnancy may have behavioural and developmental consequences. The risks associated with prenatal alcohol are greater in older mothers and in binge drinkers. Even at moderate levels (one drink per day), women who regularly consume alcohol during pregnancy may increase their risk for miscarriage or delivering low-birthweight babies.'

Chapter Five

Growing and Showing
Month Three of Pregnancy

What's going on in your body?

By Week Nine, your baby already has the start of a recognisable face: the eyes are coloured and more prominent, eyelids are visible, and there is a mouth with a tongue. Hands and feet have started to grow, with little ridges where the fingers and toes will be. And meanwhile, the internal organs – brain, heart, lungs, liver, kidneys and gut – are all developing steadily. By Week Nine, your baby will be about 22 mm (roughly the size of a sugar cube) from head to bottom. From Week Ten, your baby has officially graduated from being an 'embryo' to being a 'foetus'.

As you come to the end of your first trimester, just thirteen weeks after conception, your foetus is fully formed, with all its organs, muscles, limbs, bones and sex organs well developed. The small things are in place too: it not only has fingernails but even the first swirls of fingerprints on its fingers and thumbs! All it has to do now is concentrate on growing. It will even be moving about inside you, though you won't be able to feel it yet. You might, however, start to see a distinct bump on your tummy!

My Diary

The first work colleague to hear our news was Suzy, one of the producers of Andrew Lloyd Webber's BBC show. We got on really well and I knew I could trust her with our secret. The next series, *Over the Rainbow*, had been commissioned and filming was due to start soon, so I wanted to let everyone involved know as early as possible that I was pregnant to give them the option of whether they included me on the judging panel this time around.

I arranged for us to meet at a central London hotel, telling Suzy beforehand that it was just a social get-together so we could both get excited about the new series. But over a cup of tea I whispered to her that I was pregnant and she seemed thrilled. We had a great chat and I told her I had been wondering how it would affect my work. She reassured me that everyone would work around me, adding how special it was because I'd met Lee on an earlier series. She asked me for my permission to tell Andrew Lloyd Webber as he's obviously one of the big decision-makers, so of course I agreed. I was so pleased and couldn't have wished for the conversation to have gone any better. I left the hotel with a spring in my step, relieved that I would still be able to take part in the show I loved.

The following day I was off to interview Westlife for *Now* magazine, discussing their new album and their ten years in the business together. The boys were as lovely and cheeky as ever. During our chat I had to keep excusing myself so I could dash to the loo. It was getting a bit embarrassing. On my third return from the ladies', Shane shouted, 'Come on, Den, you're not pregnant are you?' The boys all laughed at Shane's joke so I turned around and said, 'Actually, I am.' Their jaws dropped before they all jumped up to give me a big hug, taking care not to squeeze too hard.

Shane then gave me advice on how he manages to juggle his busy career and family life (the superdad now has three kids). I admitted to him that I was worried about how becoming a mum might affect my career but he was quick to reassure me that it would have a positive effect. He went on to explain that becoming a dad had made him work even harder because he wants to provide as much as possible for his family and make his children proud.

So that was it now, the floodgates had opened, and once Westlife knew there was no keeping my secret. So immediately after the interview I sat down, phone in hand, and one by one told all of my friends (well, some got a text message or it would have taken me all year). One of the joys of getting pregnant for the first time is witnessing the happiness and excitement that your news generates amongst your friends and family, and I can honestly say that every single person I told was so thrilled for Lee and me, especially our closest friends who have known for a long time just how much we had wanted to start a family.

In less than an hour, the phone calls from the press started coming in to my publicist Simon Jones, so on his advice we released a statement confirming I was pregnant and that both Lee and I were overjoyed. That same evening I attended the *Cosmopolitan* Awards and it was such a relief to walk the red carpet, safe in the knowledge my small bump wouldn't cause speculation or gossip (is she up the duff or does she have IBS?). Even so, I opted for a dress that didn't show off my belly too much, as I was still a bit self-conscious. I know it sounds weird but I couldn't wait to be sporting a proper bump where there was no mistaking there was a baby inside. The following day the newspapers ran pictures of me from the red carpet along with the story that I was pregnant, and thankfully they were all very complimentary. From then on, people would approach Lee and me in the street to congratulate us or offer me bits of advice during my daily hot chocolate visit to Starbucks in Hampstead (aka Pramstead, as there are so many babies and young children around). We both loved that people were so happy for us.

Being pregnant just dominates everything in your life – it takes over your thought processes, your routine habits and of course most of your conversations. So it wasn't long before I realised I'd become the one thing I swore I never would be – a baby bore! And the funny thing was, I loved every minute of it. I was meeting up with my mates who already had kids and chatting for hours about motherhood. We'd cover the amazing things like seeing your baby for the first time, the first smile and the first steps, and the not-so-appealing things like the endless dirty nappies and colic. Within a matter of weeks it started to feel strange getting together with my friends who were still living the single life. As they regaled me with stories of their singleton antics, I'd sit there thinking about how I'd rather be talking about babies, whereas no more than a few months ago I'd have been right in there offering advice on how to play the field.

By now, Nicki and Amanda had adapted my diet and fitness regime to suit the early stages of pregnancy. I was really nervous about exercising at first but Nicki assured me that it was important to strike a balance between getting a decent amount of light exercise and plenty of rest. I was keen to keep up with our regular walks as already I had been getting short of breath doing the simplest things, which was down to the increase in hormones in my body. I made the silly mistake of making a work phone call while walking to the high street to pick up some milk and by the time I'd reached the end of my road I was struggling for air and having difficulty getting my words out. I must have sounded like a dirty caller with my heavy breathing. Mind you, people pay good money for that kind of thing, don't they? A career path to consider perhaps if work dries up.

From now on I was going to be avoiding any exercise too strenuous so I just continued my walks on Hampstead Heath with Nicki, occasionally staying closer to my flat when I was feeling tired. When it was raining heavily Nicki would call to cancel, because she didn't want to risk me catching a chill or slipping over on the hills.

Amanda went through my diet, stressing the importance of eating regularly throughout the day to prevent me from feeling sick. I explained that I'd been constantly craving cheese (I'd nibble on it morning, noon and night) and she advised me to eat low-fat yoghurt and ricotta cheese, as that was what my body was telling me I needed. Hey presto, as soon as I started doing this my craving disappeared, which was a relief: gigantic slabs of Cheddar at all hours were certainly contributing to my ever-increasing waistband. I find it so fascinating that your body tells you what it needs by craving different foods. Amanda also pointed out that as my immune system would be weaker than usual due to the pregnancy I needed to be sure to eat enough foods rich in nutrients such as zinc, to help protect me against all the colds that were going around. Don't get me wrong, I'm not normally the kind of person who would be worried about coughs and sneezes, but when you're in the family way the last thing you want is to be struck down by some über-bug that you're unable to shift because you can't knock back a load of Lemsip.

Something that really took me by surprise was how my taste buds changed completely. Anyone who knows me well will know the first thing I need in the morning is a nice cup of coffee, but now even so much as a whiff of it made me feel sick. I also went from being a banana-a-day girl to avoiding them altogether because I became bizarrely disgusted by their texture. At this point in my pregnancy, the way to my heart was carbs and plenty of them: shove a mountain of spag bol in front of me and it was happy days.

Having access to Amanda's expert advice was priceless and she helped me immensely, but despite my best efforts to eat the right energy-boosting foods I was becoming increasingly lethargic every day. I guess it's not surprising bearing in mind what's going on inside any pregnant lady's belly. If I was working during the day I was fit for nothing during the evening despite the valiant attempts of Lee to try and keep me awake. I could just about muster up enough energy to slather myself in any lotion or potion claiming to prevent stretch marks before slipping and sliding my way between the sheets. Poor Lee must have thought he was sleeping next to a greasy chip every night, plus he was always greeted by my back because the pregnancy books advise that you sleep on your left-hand side to allow maximum blood flow to the baby. On the occasions when he was brave enough to attempt to cuddle me, he'd either slip off or I'd have to ask him to back off to allow me to cool down or so I could make yet another trip to the loo.

A big plus side to everyone knowing I was pregnant was that people were being so understanding. At work I was getting regular breaks to rest and eat, and in my social life friends would understand if I occasionally ducked out of a get-together.

I'd been really looking forward to celebrating Kimberley Walsh's birthday with her because we'd got on so well during the Killy climb, but when the day finally arrived I was exhausted. I just couldn't face a late night at a club so I called Kimberley and was honest with her. She was really understanding; in fact she said she'd only asked me because she didn't want to leave me out, but hadn't really expected to see me there with it being such a late one. I was starting to realise that you don't have to be superwoman while you're pregnant. You have to listen to your body and just do what feels right for you.

Listening to my body was easier said than done, as one minute it was telling me it was bursting with energy and ready to face anything and then the next I'd be feeling exhausted. My constant mood swings were driving me crazy too and making me a nightmare to live with. Worst of all, I'd arrive home after working all day so depleted of energy that I was unable to clean the flat, which believe it or not is one of my favourite pastimes. Anyone who knows me will be aware of my obsession with cleanliness, which has earned me the nickname Kim Woodburn (the buxom lady who presents *How Clean Is Your House?*) – in fact my love of cleaning is bordering on OCD (not that Kim has OCD, of course). If Lee hadn't tidied up after himself when I got home I would just hit the roof. So much as a dirty plate in the wrong place would prompt the same kind of reaction you'd expect if he'd just driven a car into the living room. I'm extremely lucky he's so easy going because I was impossible to keep happy. If he *had* tidied something it wasn't done well enough or he hadn't done it the right way. I was fully aware of my erratic behaviour too, so I was constantly apologising for my outbursts after the event.

It was actually around this time I bought Myleene Klass's pregnancy book and was relieved to read she had experienced the same rollercoaster of emotions and had taken it out on her man as well. Becoming an irrational hormone monster is actually quite an upsetting transition because obviously we all care for and love our partners – who have to bear the brunt of it – but I have to admit I took great comfort in the fact it wasn't just me.

Things were going brilliantly for Lee on the work front and when he was offered the lead role in the Oscar Wilde play, *Lord Arthur Savile's Crime*, he was over the moon. It was his first major acting role and it would see him travelling around the country on tour. I could hardly blame him too if he was secretly looking forward to getting away from my constant nagging and to having his own bed at night free from the wriggling grease-beast I had now become. At first I was worried about how I was going to deal with being on my own, especially at night, but my family and friends assured me that they would be there for me. One thing we'd made clear as a couple before trying to conceive was that having a baby wouldn't interfere with Lee's career. I'm seven years older than he is and I have pretty much achieved everything I'd dreamed of and more, but Lee was just starting out and it was important to the both of us that he continued to follow his dreams, albeit now with a wife and baby waiting for him at home. Also since we got married I'd been watching the news and feeling absolute admiration for the wives of servicemen fighting in Afghanistan, who show such faith and strength when their partners are away. It helped put my concerns in context. I'd be seeing Lee at least once a week and, let's face it, Birmingham is hardly the other side of the world.

The best way for me to deal with the old man being away was to fit in as many catch-ups with friends as possible, as something told me I wouldn't be seeing them quite so regularly once the baby arrived. One evening the girls took me to see the all-singing and all-dancing movie *Nine* as they knew how much I'd been looking forward to seeing it. As we took our seats with our popcorn and drinks I reached into my bag to grab my phone. I was just reading a text message from Lee checking to see if I was OK when I felt a tap on my shoulder. I turned to see a guy glaring at me before telling me to turn my phone off. I started explaining that my phone was on silent and I was just returning a message before the film started when he shoved me really hard in my back. My friends sprung to my defence and, in the middle of what had now turned into a full-blown argument, I announced, 'I'm pregnant,' at which point everyone in the vicinity started telling the guy to leave me alone and that he was in the wrong to shove me because I was pregnant. In my opinion he was wrong to shove me, full stop. I sat physically shaking in my seat; all I could think about was the stress on the baby. The whole experience left me feeling vulnerable.

The feeling of wanting to protect my unborn child took over and, not wanting to risk getting into a similar situation, I didn't leave the house for a couple of days. But after plenty of supportive phone calls from the girls and some time to put my experience into perspective, I was back on track. In fact I did one of the best things anyone expecting their first little one could possibly do to make them feel good: I took my five-year-old niece Sophie to see the *Disney on Ice* show! She was so excited and got into the spirit of the evening by wearing her Snow White costume. Seeing all the little girls that evening dressed up as Tinkerbell, Snow White and Cinderella made me have a moment where I let myself imagine how lovely it would be to have a little girl to dress up and bake cupcakes with. She'd certainly be a mummy's girl, that's for sure.

Unfortunately, dressing *myself* wasn't quite as easy as a visit to the Disney store, and I was starting to find shopping for outfits to wear to events almost impossible. I'm sure most pregnant women who have had to dress up for a posh night out have been through the same predicament, as the choices are limited to say the least, and when you do find something that fits well and looks good it's so expensive. It was during one of those frustrating shopping trips that I decided I'd like to have a go at designing my own maternity range, and after a few well-placed phone calls that afternoon I had bagged a meeting with the team at the online fashion store Very. We met up and I explained my experience on the high street and how I'd like to design a range of maternity wear that was affordable and could be worn both during and after pregnancy. They absolutely loved the idea and within a matter of days I'd raided my wardrobe and picked out my favourite things for inspiration. Next thing I knew, the designers at Very had sent samples of the soft jersey pieces to my doorstep. I was amazed at how fast the process was and it meant I could now wear my 'Very' own range (excuse the pun) out and about, which felt fantastic.

Now for the Experts...

How exercise can help you beat fatigue

As Denise discovered, extreme fatigue is very common in the first trimester of pregnancy. Your body is hard at work creating a new life, and hormone changes, including rising levels of progesterone, can contribute to feelings of fatigue. Unfortunately people won't necessarily be making allowances for your condition as you are not visibly pregnant and you may not have told anyone yet. In addition, the emotional ups and downs of adjusting to the thought of becoming a mother can really take their toll on you at this stage.

Generally, things pick up during the second trimester, but then your energy levels will dip again during the third trimester, as you will be carrying more weight and may have more difficulty sleeping at night.

However, it's important not to give up exercising completely during pregnancy, however tired you are. The benefits are well documented: by becoming more active you will actually have *more* energy than if you succumb to the sofa (counter-intuitive as that seems), as regular exercise improves your cardiovascular system, thus increasing your energy levels. You will also suffer from fewer aches and pains and require less medical intervention during your pregnancy: studies have shown that moderate exercise can prevent varicose veins and help control gestational diabetes. Exercise will give you a healthy glow, boost your mood and give you a head start when it comes to getting your old body back after you've given birth. And not only that, but strengthening and toning your muscles will help during labour itself!

So even if it's just a brisk walk around the block, do try and get out there and do some form of light exercise *every day*, preferably in the fresh air. It will get your blood circulating, the endorphins flowing, and provide a real pick-me-up when you are flagging.

In addition, make sure you get enough rest – go to bed early, take a catnap whenever you can, buy a body pillow to help you sleep comfortably. Don't be afraid to ask for help around the house when you are absolutely exhausted. Your baby cares more about having a healthy, happy mum than having a clean kitchen floor.

Craving and going off foods in pregnancy

It is not unusual, as Denise found, to suddenly go 'off' foods and drinks that you used to love before you became pregnant. This can be a positive thing when it's something not so good for you, like coffee or alcohol.

However, even if it's something healthy – such as bananas in Denise's case – it's not something to worry about if your overall diet remains varied. Certainly bananas are 'good for you': they count towards one of your 'five a day' fruit and vegetables and are great for potassium, a mineral needed to help balance blood pressure. But so are most other fruits and vegetables, so substituting bananas with another fruit will not lead to nutritional deficiencies.

If you find yourself going off something that is otherwise a mainstay of your diet, such as milk or all dairy foods or all meat, then it is worth asking your GP if you can see a local registered dietitian who can help you find acceptable foods that will make up for the nutrients lost in your diet.

For example, if you go off meat and used to eat it regularly, then you need to find another way of getting the crucial energy-boosting mineral iron into your meals. This may mean having fortified breakfast cereals or increasing your intake of pulses and dark green vegetables.

Suddenly starting to crave foods is another frequent occurrence during pregnancy. There is a commonly held belief that we crave foods that contain nutrients that we are perhaps lacking in or need more of while pregnant.

There is not a great deal of good research in this area but it is interesting that Denise felt that her sudden desire to wolf down Cheddar was because she felt that her body needed extra calcium. If you also have cheese cravings, it is worth exploring other ways of increasing calcium in your diet, without the weight gain associated with high-fat cheese. For example you could add extra skimmed milk to drinks like decaffeinated lattes, seek out 0% fat yoghurts and include other calcium-rich foods such as sesame seeds and dark green vegetables in your diet.

Turning to single-nutrient supplements is not a good idea unless you do so on the advice of your GP or health visitor. This is because having too much of one vitamin or mineral can cause an imbalance in the absorption and use of another in your body. Stick to multivitamins specially designed for pregnant women.

Craving non-food items during pregnancy is known as *pica* and refers to the desire to eat things like soil, ice or ash. If you find yourself in the grip of pica, you must talk with your doctor or midwife and get their advice.

The good news about pregnancy cravings is that they tend to diminish from the third month.

Chapter Six

Pink or Blue?
Month Four of Pregnancy

What's going on in your body?

You're now at the beginning of your second trimester, in other words the second third of your pregnancy. The great news is that things get easier again in this trimester: you'll be proudly sporting a neat bump but you won't yet be huge; you should start having more energy again; any morning sickness should have passed (with luck); and by this time the worst danger of miscarriage is over so you can start to relax on that front too. You may even notice your hair getting thicker and shinier and your skin looking more radiant as you get that pregnancy 'bloom'! On the negative side, you may start suffering from stretch marks, swollen feet and the constant need to pee as your rapidly expanding uterus starts pressing up against your bladder.

As for your baby, by Week Fourteen it will be about 8½ cm from head to bottom (roughly the size of an apple), increasing to around 12½ to 14 cm by the end of Week Seventeen. Its head will gradually start to uncurl, so it no longer rests on its chest. Eyebrows and eyelashes are growing, and by the end of the month it will be able to hiccup and swallow. From about Week Seventeen onwards, you might just be able to feel your baby move inside you, though it will be more of a light fluttering or bubbling sensation than a kick at this stage.

My Diary

We were just four weeks away from our twenty-week scan now, which offered us the opportunity of finding out the sex of the ever-growing bump we kept referring to as 'it'. Lee and I had many discussions about whether or not we'd like to know and we soon found out that it's another of those pregnancy topics that everyone has an opinion on. 'It spoils the surprise on the day of the birth'; 'we couldn't tell in my day so you shouldn't find out'; 'there'll be no reason to push if you already know the sex' – these were just a few of the reasons given to us as to why we shouldn't find out. After weighing up all of the pros and cons we came to the conclusion that we *did* want to find out. For me, going to our twenty-week scan and not finding out the sex would be like saving the delicious chocolate bar in the fridge for a rainy day – it was never going to happen.

We had already decided on a name for each sex, so we felt that finding out would help us to bond with 'it' and we could start choosing the little extras that define a boy's or a girl's nursery. I love interior design and had been looking forward to getting stuck into the nursery for ages. As Lee was on tour with his play, he could pick up a few bits and pieces while he was on his travels without having to opt for neutral colours.

By now I was pretty much convinced we were having a boy anyway because nearly everyone around me kept telling me that was what I was having. It's funny how, when you're pregnant, complete strangers come up to you in the street or in the freezer section of Sainsbury's to tell you what they think the sex of your baby is, just because of the way you look or how you are carrying your bump. After close inspection of my stomach and backside some would tell me I was having a boy because I was carrying low, while others would be convinced it was a boy because I hadn't suffered terribly from morning sickness and was looking well in general. My trainer Nicki was the only person who was adamant I was having a girl. Of course it really didn't matter: Lee and I, like most parents-to-be, would be happy either way as long as our bundle of joy was healthy.

Along with the sex predictions from everyone I was now receiving plenty of useful advice on pregnancy and impending motherhood: weird and wonderful methods to get the baby into a sleep routine; the best prams to get around hilly Hampstead; exhortations to get as much sleep as possible whenever you can. That was one particular piece of advice I was keen to adhere to. However, no information felt more valuable to me at this point than the updates from my friend Karen, who had just given birth to baby Rose. I was itching to visit as soon as possible to meet her and to remind myself just how tiny a newborn baby really is.

I left it a couple of weeks before I popped round to visit to allow them time to settle in, but I had the shock of my life when Karen opened the door. My usually glamorous mate stood there looking a shadow of her former self, with Brian May hair and her body swamped in a baggy t-shirt and leggings. Her husband Dave didn't look any fresher, sporting an unshaven face and dark-circled eyes. One thing was obvious – these guys hadn't had a decent night's kip in ages.

Inside, the living room resembled the aftermath of an all-night party. There were candles burning around the room, the sofa was piled high with cushions and the curtains were still drawn. Think gothic teenager's bedroom. It was a complete contrast to my visit just a few weeks earlier when I remember thinking how organised

Karen seemed. The nursery was decked out in a pretty vintage theme and everything had its place; nappies, wipes and baby grows were all in a neat order; she had thought of everything and I had nothing but admiration for her. Quite frankly, seeing her now scared me. What had I let myself in for?

Over some biscuits and a cup of tea (that I insisted on making), she filled me in on everything. The birth was incredible but absolutely exhausting, and since arriving home she hadn't had the chance to catch up. The reality was that Rose needed feeding constantly and she felt as if she'd been living on the sofa virtually day and night (that'd explain the Eiffel Tower of cushions). Although Karen expected motherhood to be hard work there was apparently no preparation for it being so draining. I assured her that this tended to be a standard feeling among all of my friends who have had children while I quietly panicked inside.

Karen confessed to me that she had only answered a handful of important phone calls since Rose had been born and her voicemail box was full with messages from friends congratulating her and wondering when they could visit. She just wasn't feeling ready to speak to people, let alone welcome visitors to the house. It was an invaluable insight into the reality of motherhood and how I might be feeling when my time came, so I decided to pre-warn people and let them know not to worry if they didn't hear from me straight away after I'd given birth, as I was probably just getting used to being a mum.

At last Rose finally woke up. At 7 lbs 7 oz she was the youngest and smallest baby I had ever held. As I cuddled her she felt so delicate that I was afraid to move her too much in case I broke or squashed her. She was just so gorgeous and teeny tiny that I couldn't quite believe it.

With most new mothers, once you look past the initial veneer of chaos and fatigue it becomes clear that actually everything's under control, and Karen was no exception. As I watched her she looked every bit the natural mother; I could see the confident way she held her precious little bundle of joy, changed her and comforted her. I asked her how she knew what to do and she assured me that my instincts would kick in once my little one arrived. I sincerely hoped so but I wasn't convinced. After I got home the doubts about whether I was actually ready became overwhelming.

That night I had another episode of what had become a recurring dream: I would be out in a public place and I'd suddenly drop my newborn baby. Everyone would be looking over, pointing at me, and a few would rush to my aid, but I'd be in such a panic I'd be unable to move. In this particular dream I was in Sainsbury's, holding the baby in one arm and steering the trolley with the other. I reached up to get something from the top shelf and dropped the baby. Everyone started panicking and I was frantically looking around for help, when my mum ran over out of nowhere yelling, 'What have you done?' I was devastated. As per usual I woke up in the morning feeling really freaked out. I couldn't help thinking I wasn't ready to become a mum, even my dreams were telling me so.

The night before our twenty-week scan, Lee and I just sat up chatting for hours, unable to sleep with the familiar excitement that preceded any of our scans, let alone the one that would tell us whether we'd be opting for pink or blue décor in the nursery.

So the next day, I lay there on the bed as the sonographer Dr Pran did the scan (I really looked forward to walking into the hospital and telling the receptionist I was there for a scan with Pran). Swiftly, he located the baby's heartbeat and, as usual, seeing it beat away fifteen to the dozen brought a tear to my eye. As he then checked all of the measurements I was just dying to ask so many questions. It's always worrying when the person checking the health of your baby goes silent but I figured it would be best to keep quiet myself and let him concentrate on the job at hand. With the serious stuff out of the way he dropped the big question: would we like to know the sex of our baby? A quick glimpse across to Lee prompted him to confirm, 'Yes, we'd love to.' Another squirt of cold gel smeared onto my belly, a quick manoeuvre of the scanner and he announced, 'Well, I'm pleased to tell you you're having a baby girl.' It had barely registered with me when Lee punched the air with a big 'Yes!' as if he'd just scored a winning penalty.

A girl? I was confused. I was so convinced we were having a boy – everyone had been telling me so. I asked whether he was completely sure and if he'd mind taking another look. He gave me a wry smile and said, 'I've been doing this a very long time and you're definitely having a girl.' To put my mind at rest he pointed to three white lines on the screen and said, 'That's the female genitalia just there.'

We were on our way home from the hospital when Lee admitted that – despite thinking we were having a boy and both of us saying we didn't mind either way – he had secretly hoped for a girl all along. I hadn't expected finding out the sex of our baby to have such a big effect on him, but he was ecstatic that he was going to have a daughter and to be honest with you so was I. Those guilty daydreams of making cupcakes and playing dress-up would now become reality.

Despite being in a state of disbelief and still wondering whether there was any chance the doctor had got it wrong, we set about calling all our family and friends to tell them the news. Of course most of them were as shocked as we were, having thought there was a little boy on the way.

As I mentioned earlier, we'd previously gone through the name selection process so our little girl already had her name, but rather than reveal it to everyone we decided to keep it to ourselves until she was born, so we had something between just Lee and myself. Besides, one of my friends had the worst-case scenario when she told everyone the name she'd decided on for her little girl only to find that one of her acquaintances had pinched it for her baby who was born a few days earlier than hers. Who would have thought choosing the name would be so political? We'd also been warned that she may not look like the name we had for her when we saw her for the first time, and some friends suggested we made a short list of alternatives just in case. Now that's a bizarre statement to me – surely you grow into the name you're given rather than the other way round? I don't understand how people can say, 'Ah, she looks like a Pamela,' or 'Oh, I think she's more of a Sheila,' when looking at a newborn baby.

In any case, Lee and I made a solemn promise not to tell anyone, though the only trouble was that Lee kept slipping up by accidentally calling the bump by her name in front of friends. A sharp kick under the table usually stopped him in mid-flow but, bless him, his bruised shins must have been painful. We were going to need a codename.

Now for the Experts...

You should have a little more energy in this trimester, so it's a good time to review your fitness regime and perhaps gently increase your efforts. This is the month when all the benefits will start to pay off. Bear in mind your body is growing and changing all the time, so it's more important than ever that you invest in a well-fitting support bra in which to exercise – and be aware you may need a new one before your pregnancy is over as your boobs continue to grow!

As your uterus starts to expand rapidly this month, you will also need to remember not to lie on your back for periods longer than two to three minutes, either when you're exercising or when you're at rest. There's a risk the baby may lie on the blood vessels leading to the placenta, and cut off its food and oxygen supply.

Continue with your pregnancy exercise regime as outlined in Chapter One, or maybe use your newfound energy to investigate doing something you've not tried before, such as yoga, perhaps?

Prenatal yoga

These days, yoga is one of the most popular ways to exercise in pregnancy. Why? Well, its mix of strengthening, balancing, stretching, relaxation and breathing is an excellent way to tone your muscles, increase your stamina and lung capacity, improve your circulation and digestion, and become more connected with your body. The breathing and relaxation techniques found in yoga even help prepare for labour, and many of the squatting positions help to strengthen and open the pelvic floor muscles. Yoga can also help you maintain good posture throughout your pregnancy because it focuses on core, back and shoulder strength.

With its focus on deep breathing, yoga has a uniquely calming quality that can help you during the turbulent emotional changes of pregnancy. It's also a great way to meet other mums-to-be in a nurturing, relaxed environment.

All that said, it's best to join a special pregnancy yoga class if possible (or use a prenatal yoga DVD), or at the least make sure you have told your regular teacher you are pregnant and ensure they are fully trained in what you can and can't do. You won't be able to do poses that require you to lie on your back or stomach, for example, and you should be wary about doing inverted poses or deep twists from the belly if they are uncomfortable. Remember you are more flexible when pregnant due to the hormone relaxin, so you are more at risk of injury due to overdoing it. Avoid jumping moves and skip any exercises that require you to hold your breath or perform a succession of rapid inhales and exhales.

There are various different types of yoga, each with its own special focus and level of intensity. With the exception of Bikram, yoga is generally considered safe and beneficial for women during pregnancy. See overleaf for a guide to different yoga styles.

Ashtanga

This is a powerful, flowing form of yoga suitable for experienced practitioners or the very fit. It focuses on strength, flexibility and stamina.

Bikram

This is a very physical and intense form of yoga that is performed in a room heated to at least 105 degrees Fahrenheit. It can help reduce symptoms of disease and chronic pain by focusing on twenty-six postures performed in a specific order. Bikram should only be attempted by very fit individuals: pregnant women should not practise this type of yoga.

Couples' Yoga

This is becoming increasingly popular, working to bring couples together and improving communication and interconnectivity as they perform the positions together.

Hatha (incorporating Iyengar yoga)

This is a very common type of yoga. Gentle and flowing, it focuses on simple poses, deep breathing, meditation and improved posture. It is perfect for beginners or those who haven't exercised in a while, and uses props such as straps, blocks and pillows to compensate for limited flexibility.

Kripalu

This is another gentle variant of yoga. Through a series of flowing postures, it aims to increase awareness of the mind, body, and spirit. It has a strong meditative aspect.

Kundalini

Incorporating chanting, meditation, visualisations, and guided relaxation, kundalini yoga focuses on healing and purifying the mind, body and emotions.

Sivananda

Consisting of twelve poses that incorporate breathing, relaxation, and mantra chanting, this is another of the most popular forms of yoga.

Viniyoga

Viniyoga is a slower, more personalised form of yoga that develops strength, balance, and healing. It is ideal for beginners, seniors, people with chronic pain or who are rehabilitating from injury or disease.

Yoga stretches to try at home

If you are interested in trying out yoga but don't want to commit to a class, on the next pages are a few gentle poses you can try at home.

Note: *As the first two poses involve lying on your back, you may want to skip them in late pregnancy – in any case, do not hold the position for more than two minutes once you are in the second trimester or beyond.*

Supported Bridge Pose

1 Lie on your back with your knees bent and your feet flat on the floor. Walk your feet back so they are positioned as close to your buttocks as possible.

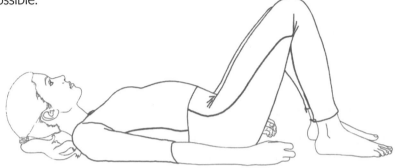

2 Inhale and exhale, and then slowly raise your pelvis and buttocks off the floor, while keeping your thighs and inner feet parallel.

3 Clasp your hands behind your back underneath you.

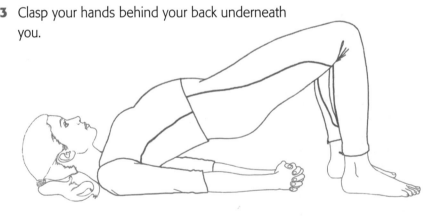

4 Hold this pose, while breathing deeply, for no more than one or two minutes if you are in the second trimester or beyond.

Legs on the Wall Pose

1 Lie on your side on the floor with your bottom close to a wall. You may want to place a rolled towel or blanket under your neck for support.

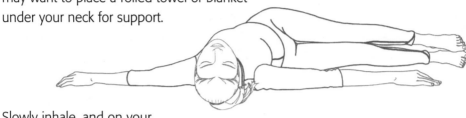

2 Slowly inhale, and on your exhale, rotate your body and lie on your back so that your legs move up and rest upside-down against the wall. You want to create a ninety-degree angle at your pelvis.

3 Hold for no more than two minutes if you are in the second trimester or beyond, and then release your legs slowly.

Cobbler's Pose

1 Sit on the floor with your legs stretched out straight in front of you. Try not to let your back slouch.
2 Inhale, and slowly move your feet towards your groin, pushing the soles of your feet together.
3 While exhaling, gently lower your knees towards the ground while holding on to your toes. Try not to let your leg muscles strain too much.
4 Hold this posture for between one and five minutes.

Eating to beat constipation in pregnancy

Although the second trimester generally heralds a new period of increased wellbeing for the mum-to-be, there are still some common niggles during this time from which you may be suffering. One such problem is constipation, which affects almost forty per cent of women in the UK during their pregnancies. It is believed in part to be triggered by a slowing up of the speed at which the intestines normally work, which means that waste is not pushed through as quickly and therefore becomes a bit stuck and hard to pass. It's also thought that during pregnancy our bodies absorb more fluid from the large intestine, resulting in less water in the stools, which in turn makes them harder and more difficult to push out. A third reason is the fact that simply being less physically active can increase the problem, since exercise helps to keep the gut working well. Finally, if you have been given iron supplements to help reverse an iron deficiency, these too may be having a 'binding' effect.

The good news is that there are simple changes you can make to your diet that can help with this problem – indeed, earlier on in Denise's pregnancy she mentions that eating a healthier diet had helped to 'make her regular' in the bathroom department. It's certainly worth doing everything you can to beat constipation as not only is it unpleasant in itself, but it can also be a contributing factor to the development of piles, another common pregnancy ailment. Try to make the dietary changes listed below as soon as you can, as in a survey one-fifth of women questioned said that the last three months were the worst for this problem. So start following these guidelines now!

✳ While pregnant, try to get your **fibre intake** up to around 27 g per day. At the moment the average UK intake is about 12 g although the recommended target in normal day-to-day life is 18 g. All wholegrain foods, such as wholemeal bread, wholegrain breakfast cereals, brown pasta, pitta bread and rice, give us good amounts of fibre. Vegetables and fruits are useful too, especially raspberries, dried figs, baked beans and other pulses.

❋ Drink plenty of **water**. While there is no really solid scientific evidence to say that drinking water makes your stools softer and easier to pass, it is widely recommended by health professionals such as registered dietitans and registered nutritionists whose advice is to 'drink plenty of water daily'. Try drinking a few extra glasses of water with and between meals.

❋ Eat **prunes**. It is old advice, but good advice. Prunes contain sorbitol, a natural sugar-alcohol (nothing to do with the alcohol you drink!) that helps to hurry up your intestines and relieve constipation. If you don't like the idea of them on things like cereal or in winter fruit salads (made of dried fruits), then try canned ones that have been drained and blitzed into a smoothie with yoghurt and banana or other fruits you fancy.

❋ Eat **sugar-free sweets**. These contain other natural sugar-alcohols such as lacitol and manitol. They all have the effect of speeding up the intestine and can help to prevent or treat constipation. Half a small packet of sugar-free sweets should do the trick.

❋ When buying processed foods, look for those with more than 6 g of fibre per 100 g (or the portion you can reasonably be expected to eat in a normal day). If a food has 6 g of fibre or more in this amount then it is a **'high fibre' food** and is well worth putting in your basket – if it not also bursting with fat and sugar, that is!

Eating to beat swollen ankles in pregnancy

One other common niggle in pregnancy that might start to strike in the second trimester is swollen ankles. Denise started suffering from this problem around this time, and it commonly gets worse as the pregnancy goes on. You may also notice, like Denise, that your hands are affected too, with rings getting tighter and uncomfortable as a result.

The good news is that, in most women, this common 'side-effect' of pregnancy is annoying but not dangerous. It occurs because of the increase in the amount of blood in your body while pregnant. As your baby grows bigger in your womb, it puts pressure on the blood vessels in your pelvis and slows the circulation of blood back to the heart. This causes the blood to pool and forces water from your blood out through tiny capillaries and into the tissues in your feet, ankles or fingers.

Although common, it is still important that you talk to your midwife or GP about any swelling because in a small number of women it can be a sign of another problem such as pre-eclampsia or deep-vein thrombosis, both of which can be serious for you and your baby. If the swelling happens very quickly and causes headaches, pain in the stomach, confusion, shortness of breath, blurred or altered vision, nausea or vomiting and simply feeling unwell, you must get medical help right away.

For women who are experiencing uncomplicated swelling and have been given the all-clear by a health professional, then following some simple tips may help to relieve the problem.

✳ Try to **avoid processed foods** that are often rich in salt, as this can make water retention worse. A diet that is fairly low in salt should help to keep blood pressure within normal parameters as well. Eating the foods suggested in Chapter One should help you to achieve a cut in your normal salt intakes, but the number-one piece of advice is to avoid as much processed food as possible because seventy-five per cent of our salt intake comes from things like certain breakfast cereals, ready-made soups, ready meals and fast food.

* When shopping, look for foods that have **less than 0.3 g salt** (or 0.1 g of sodium) per serving or per 100 g . These foods can legitimately claim to be low salt. Those with more than 1.3 g of salt per serving or per 100 g (or 0.5 g of sodium) contain a lot of salt and are probably best avoided where possible.

* Don't take **diuretics** when you are pregnant.

* Try to keep your feet **elevated** whenever possible and if you get a chance to lie down, take it!

* **Support tights** may help, but only wear them on the advice of your GP.

* **Gentle exercise** like swimming and walking may also help to keep your blood flowing as efficiently as possible.

Chapter Seven

Who Ate All the Mince Pies?
Month Five of Pregnancy

What's going on in your body?

At around Week Eighteen, your baby starts to become covered in a fine, soft hair called 'lanugo'. No one quite knows why this happens, but it's thought it helps to keep the baby at the right temperature. (Don't worry, it mainly disappears over the next couple of months so you won't be giving birth to a monkey!) Your baby's hearing is not yet mature but it will still be able to hear you and begin to recognise your voice. Its growth rate will slow a little from now on, but it will still continue to gain weight constantly.

Week Twenty is a big milestone as you'll have now officially reached the halfway point in your pregnancy. (Though don't get too excited: remember it's only actually been eighteen weeks since conception and you've still got twenty to go…) Most women will be offered a scan around this point, when they can determine the sex of their baby if they choose. By now, your baby will be about 16 cm long from top of head to bottom (the size of a cantaloupe melon), and weigh about 280 g. Not bad considering it was just a tiny bundle of cells eighteen weeks ago!

My Diary

Now I'm no princess and the pea, believe me, but I do like my nice cosy bed for preferably eight hours of uninterrupted sleep. Unfortunately, my bump had a different idea altogether of how much sleep I should be getting. Having now reached an awkward size, it was becoming increasingly uncomfortable to lie in bed. Morphing into a giant whale combined with searing hot flushes and a ridiculous number of loo trips meant I was lucky if I slept three hours straight. In fact I'd often get up in the morning feeling like I hadn't slept at all, so with the image of Karen still permanently etched into my mind I'd sneak a couple of extra hours under the duvet whenever I could. Fortunately my diary had eased off a little as the entertainment industry tends to wind down towards the end of November, so for me this was the perfect time to catch up with friends and family. I'm such a huge fan of Christmas that my festive spirit usually kicks in from the first of December, so I was ready for some serious down-time and mulled wine (the latter I'd have to forgo myself unfortunately). Of course this year was going to be different; Lee and I had less than five months until our baby girl arrived, so it would be our last footloose and fancy-free Christmas before we'd have a little person to worry about and fuss over.

Despite the constant fatigue I was determined to enjoy the festivities and indulge in my favourite Christmas pastime, shopping for the kids. A few of my close friends who have experienced first-hand what I'm like when I hit the high street tried to persuade me it would be a better idea to shop online, with my feet up in the comfort of my own home. But that's not what it's all about for me. While most people find it a chore to battle around the high street, I love the hustle and bustle of Oxford Street over the festive period.

Give me carol singers, Christmas lights and hot chocolate and I'm in my element, so despite my friends' best efforts I opted for the real thing.

There are so many children in my family and circle of friends that a few years ago I made a rule that the adults receive token gifts for Christmas whereas the kids get spoilt, so each year I spend hours blissfully wandering around children's departments playing with the latest toys and games like I'm in a scene from the famous Tom Hanks movie, *Big*.

My six-year-old niece Sophie is always fun to buy for as she loves all things girly. If two words could sum up her toy cupboard they would be 'fairy' and 'princess', but this year was even more special for me because I could now imagine playing with all the toys with my very own little princess. How exciting.

My seven-year-old nephews, Cameron and Sunny, aren't quite so easy to shop for as I'm not so clued up on the latest action figures for little boys (if ever you can be clued up; they tend to change every five minutes). A call to my brother Terry didn't help as he may as well have been talking Chinese when he started reeling off a list of action figures I'd never heard of. When I asked him to slow down he laughed before telling me, 'Trust me, sis, this time next year you'll not only know all the characters but you'll be singing the theme tunes too.' A different kind of show tune to what I'm used to but I'll no doubt give it my all. In fact with both Lee and I as parents, I was pretty sure our baby would be treated to her very own musical productions.

With the kids' presents finally sorted, I treated myself and Bump to a well-earned early Christmas present: a giant pillow. Oh, how glam! After talking to my girlfriends who have also been on this journey of back pain and restless nights, they all advised me to invest in a good nursing pillow. These were a new concept to me so shopping for one was somewhat educational as I discovered they come in all different shapes and sizes. After road-testing them (well, more like wrestling them), I settled for a giant half moon-shaped thing. It was a revelation and instantly became my best friend, taking the strain off my back when I was sitting on the sofa and off my belly while lying in bed. I can't recommend them enough.

I didn't even bat an eyelid as I continued up the escalator in John Lewis, past the second-floor designer gear where I used to while away many an hour. This time last year I would have been tempted by a sassy little pair of Jimmy Choo shoes, but right now all I cared about was whether my shoes could accommodate my swollen ankles. I felt more at home than ever on the fourth floor amongst the parents and kids, thinking that'll be me and my little girl next year.

As I was either Christmas shopping or hoofing it between meetings, I was finding it impossible to muster up any extra energy to exercise with Nicki. I explained to her how I was feeling, expecting her to adapt my exercise schedule, but she told me I was doing enough and to be careful not to overdo it. Shopping and walking from A to B is the kind of exercise you don't actually realise you're doing but it's important to take into account when you're pregnant so you don't overdo it and get run down. A healthy immune system in a city in winter is absolutely essential because there are so many coughs and colds going around. I decided it was far better for me to walk around town wrapped up warm than to sit on a tube in the firing line of germs.

Outside I was loving the weather, especially as it had started to snow, making it feel even more Christmassy. However, inside my flat I was having a constant battle with the thermostat. I just couldn't get the temperature right – the gauge was up and down as I went from hot to cold within minutes. In the end I found the best solution was to keep the heating on full blast and have the windows open. Passers-by must have thought I was mad, but how else was I supposed to cope with the rollercoaster ride of hormonal hot flushes? As for poor Lee, he was wrapped up like an Artic explorer.

By now it was mid-December, and to really get into the Christmas spirit my mate Sam and I took our nieces to see Father Christmas at Selfridges before heading to the huge Winter Wonderland Christmas fair which is held in London's Hyde Park each year. Of course I had to give the bumper cars and rollercoaster a miss, but it was so lovely to watch the two girls shriek with laughter as they tried all the rides, their eyes flicking about from one set of bright lights to the next as they walked around holding hands and giggling. With Sam's younger sister Nikki having two little girls and me with one on the way it seemed the perfect opportunity to persuade Sam she needed to join the mummy club too, so we spent most of the evening trying to convince her that if there was ever a right time this was it. I don't think she knew what hit her that night but I was a convert and wanted everyone to join my new club.

On Christmas day, Lee and I played host to our families, well for half of the day anyway. I did my bit preparing and then promptly devouring the Christmas lunch before flaking out on the sofa. This was a momentous occasion for me because it was the first time I had ever beaten my dad to the sofa for a snooze. He was most unimpressed, bless him, but I was a girl in need. It was the faint rustle of Quality Street being unwrapped that finally brought me around in time to join in the exchanging of presents. This year we had asked for things for the baby so it was really exciting to be opening bottle sterilisers, babygros and blankets, as weird as that may sound.

A few days chilling out at home and I was ready for our girly Christmas get-together with Anna and Cockney Vik, but this time instead of feeling down and questioning what life was all about, I felt like the cat that had got the cream with everyone fussing around me and congratulating me in person. Cockney Vik was so pleased that her daughter Annabel would now have a playmate to balance out Anna's two boisterous boys. Annabel, who is the loveliest little girl with the cheekiest smile, was paying special attention to my bump. 'Have you got a baby growing in your belly?' she asked, to which I replied, 'Yes I have, and she's a girl like you.' Her face lit up. 'What's her name?' was her next question, which put me in an awkward position because of course Lee and I had promised to keep it between ourselves. I pretended we hadn't chosen one yet and asked her if she could help me out. She looked straight at my bump as if it was going to magically reveal a name to her before looking back up at me and saying, 'Teapot'. We all fell about laughing but she was deadly serious. I explained to Annabel that I'd have to run the name past Lee, who absolutely adores her, so I gave him a quick call and of course he agreed that our bump would be named Teapot from then on.

New Year's Eve was a family affair once again and saw the Van Outen clan descend on the London's West End *en masse* to see *The Lion King*, which is just the most amazing and uplifting show. Still singing 'Hakuna Matata', we headed back to our flat in north London so we could see in the New Year in a slightly calmer environment than central London. Normally, for some bizarre reason, we end up singing 'Auld Lang Syne' early, which has become a bit of a running joke in our household, so this year I put the TV on full blast so we could all hear the countdown properly, and as I watched all the revellers on the bank of the River Thames part of me wished we were there in the thick of it all.

Just before midnight Lee turned to me and said, 'This year is going to be amazing; this is the year our baby girl will be born.' I'd like to tell you he then kissed me while putting a loving hand on Teapot, making it the perfect start to 2010, but what actually happened was far from romantic. With my dad in the garden, poised ready to light the fireworks he'd been meticulously plotting to rival the display down at the Thames, my mum started shouting for everyone to hurry to the garden before midnight. My little niece Sophie, who had been dancing around the lounge with excitement, made a mad dash for the back door but tripped on the way and flew through the doorway, landing with a loud thud on the patio. We all stood there for a few seconds registering what had just happened before: Five, four, three, two… 'Waaaaahhhhhh!' Wails of pain rang through the air, louder than any screaming rocket, just as Big Ben struck midnight. Lee took my hand and we gave each other a knowing smile. We had it all to come.

Now for the Experts...

Due to her Christmas shopping exploits, Denise got most of her exercise in this month from walking. It's not to be overlooked: regular walking is a great way to exercise during pregnancy, as it is so safe and gets you out in the fresh air. But if it's too cold or rainy to face going outside, there is another very low-impact form of exercise that is perfect for pregnancy and that is swimming.

As we mentioned in Chapter One, swimming is great news for pregnant women as it takes your weight off your legs and back – particularly important in this trimester as your tummy will be growing at a rate of knots and you will be feeling increasingly heavy. Aqua aerobics will help you tone up without exposing you to the risk of injury, as your body is so supported by the water, and swimming itself will help burn fat and improve your cardiovascular fitness levels. Many people find it a great way to relax too: there is something about being in water that is very soothing, as those opting for a water-birth would agree. And if you are prone to hot flushes during pregnancy, as Denise was, then swimming is a good way to exercise without overheating.

If you don't fancy joining a class or there isn't one near you, you can still get a good water workout (which doesn't involve you ploughing up and down the pool for hours), simply by following the routine below on your own. You don't even need to be able to swim to do this.

Start by warming up for five minutes or so, either by swimming a few laps or walking a few widths of the pool in the shallow end. Then alternate aerobic activity such as walking or jogging across the pool, with low-intensity recovery periods. Start with fifteen seconds of each and increase as long as you continue to feel comfortable. Repeat this high–low interval for three minutes, then try one of the strengthening moves outlined below. Follow this with another aerobic set and then another strengthening move, continuing for a full thirty-minute workout. When you have finished, cool down for five minutes by swimming some laps or walking around the pool, and do a few gentle stretches before getting out.

Remember to drink plenty of water while you are exercising, even though you may not feel like you are sweating, and never jump or dive into the pool. If you are in an outside pool somewhere hot (lucky you!), apply plenty of sunscreen and avoid the hottest times of the day (between ten in the morning and three in the afternoon) as your skin can be more sun-sensitive during pregnancy. As with all forms of exercise during pregnancy, stop if you experience any of the warning signs mentioned on page 50.

Strengthening moves in the pool

* Stand in the shallow end of the pool facing the stairs. Slowly step up onto the lowest rung, and then back down. Repeat ten times leading with one leg, then ten times leading with the other. Next turn sideways so the steps are on your right and again step up ten times, leading with your right leg. Turn and face the other way and repeat using your left leg. Finally, stand with the steps behind you and step up backwards ten times on each leg. You may need to hold on to the bar to your side for balance, but don't use your arms to pull yourself up.

* This is a good strengthening move for your arms and chest. Hold a float upright in front of you using both hands, so it's up on one end and immersed halfway in the water. Walk from one side of the pool to the other while pushing the float in front of you, using the water's resistance. Try to keep the board straight. Turn around and walk back again, zig-zagging the board in front of you.

* Stand with your back flat against the edge of the pool, with your elbows supporting you on the rim. Keeping your knees straight, slowly bring both legs up to a ninety-degree angle in front of you and hold them there for ten seconds while exhaling slowly. Then bend at the knee to bring your legs down, and repeat as many times as you're able. Be sure to keep your back straight throughout this exercise.

* The dolphin kick is a good all-round toning exercise if you can swim underwater: put your face down into the water, keep your arms by your sides and legs together, and propel yourself forward by rolling your body down from your head. Imagine a wave travelling down your body. Your legs will naturally want to separate but try to keep them together. If you find it difficult, try holding a float in front of you. You may feel more like an ungainly whale than a sleek dolphin at first, but you will improve with practice.

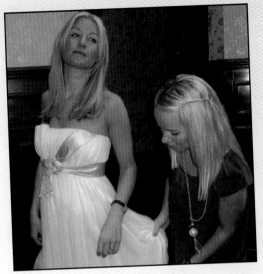

The final fitting for my wedding dress. No more chips for me until after the big day.

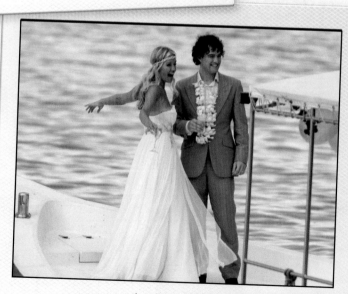

Just married and have never been happier.

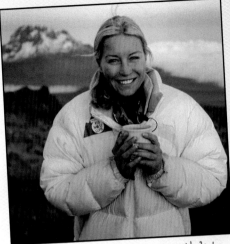

Even at the top of Kilimanjaro I couldn't be without my PG Tips.

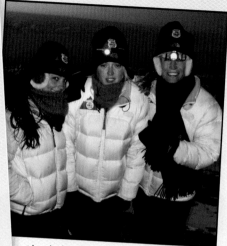

My climbing partners Cheryl Cole and Fearne Cotton. I know we look stupid but it was minus 20!

First baby for Denise the ladette and her Lee

By Elisa Roche
Showbusiness Editor

DENISE Van Outen and husband Lee Mead are expecting their first child, they confirmed yesterday.

The 35-year-old actress and TV presenter is 14 weeks pregnant and the couple, pictured right, are "delighted" at the news.

"Denise and Lee can't wait to start their family," said a spokesman.

Denise and Mead, 28, met on the BBC talent show Any Dream Will Do, when she appeared as a judge.

Mead said to win the prize – a starring role in the West End relaunch of Joseph And The Amazing Technicolour Dreamcoat.

The couple, who began dating after the show, married in a private ceremony on a beach in the Seychelles in April.

Mead said earlier this year: "Marriage for me is for life, and life with Denise is fantastic.

"We've moved into a country pile in Kent, complete with sheep! I'd love to have children and hope we can start a family. It's a really exciting time."

Ladette Denise presented The Big Breakfast on Channel 4 alongside Johnny Vaughan and went on to star in the musical Chicago in London's West End and on Broadway in New York.

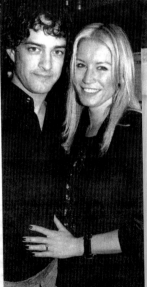

'Tis the season to be jolly fat for mum-to-be Van Outen

WEST END star Denise Van Outen is not taking pregnancy lying down. Yesterday, the first-time mother-to-be was manning a stall at a car-boot sale — although, admittedly, it was for charity and at Selfridges.

The actress and TV presenter, who announced she was 14 weeks pregnant last week, was happy to be involved in the lively shoppers' crush.

"It's like I've been waiting my whole life to be pregnant," says Denise, 35, who married Lee Mead, 28 – the winner of the Any Dream Will Do TV show — in the Seychelles in April.

"I'm doing and checking all the things that I've always thought were necessary. For instance, I sit down a lot on the assumption my ankles are swollen, but they're not.

"I'm overfeeding myself all the most sugary items from the cupboard, despite not yet having any cravings for them. I've also already been on the lookout for big pavlova-type clothes, though I can still fit into my looser items at home.

"It's all a bit of an experience. Jokes aside, I'm extremely excited about the months ahead and I'm looking forward — for the first time in my life — to looking fat for a real reason."

Denise was joined by Yasmin Le Bon, Tamara Beckwith and Jodie Kidd, who were all selling their old clothes for NSPCC Merseykids/Children.

ANY PRAM WILL DO

Baby's on the way for TV Denise and Joseph hunk

By Rick Fulton
reporters@dailyrecord.co.uk

TELLY star Denise Van Outen is expecting her first child, she revealed yesterday.

The 35-year-old – who is married to West End star Lee Mead – is 14 weeks pregnant.

The couple met when she was judging Andrew Lloyd Webber's talent show Any Dream Will Do, which Lee won.

Yesterday, their spokesman said: "Both she and Lee are absolutely delighted and can't wait to start their family."

The couple's romance started in 2007 when they met on the BBC's hunt for the lead for Webber's revival of Joseph And The Amazing Technicolor Dreamcoat.

THRILLED: Denise with husband Lee

DENISE PRAM OUTEN

TELLY host Denise Van Outen is pregnant with her first child, The Sun can reveal.

Denise, 35 — once linked to David Walliams — had her 12-week scan this week.

She and hubby Lee Mead, 28, spent last night singing for joy and pals to break the news.

A source said: "To say they are ecstatic would be an understatement. The baby's healthy and everything's going to plan."

Denise is due to give birth in May — just at the climax of

EXCLUSIVE by GORDON SMART

her new show to find a Wizard Of Oz stage star. A pal said: "She's insisting she'll work all through her pregnancy."

Denise met Lee when she was a judge on BBC's Any Dream Will Do talent show.

She was previously said to have made a bizarre marriage pact with Walliams. The pair agreed in 2006 that they would wed each other within two years if neither had found love.

Expecting . . . Denise and hubby Lee

Ex . . star out with Walliams in 2005

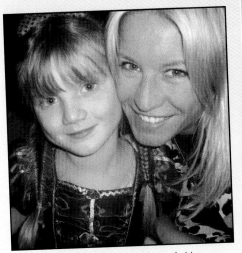

Disney on Ice at the O2 Arena. Ah bless – my niece Sophie in her Snow White costume.

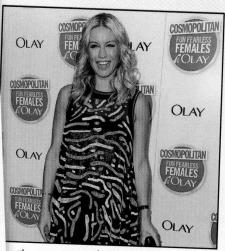

The Cosmo Awards – relieved that I could finally tell everyone I was pregnant.

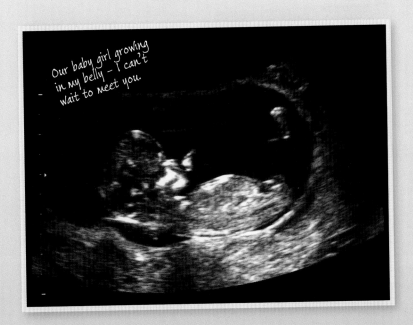

Our baby girl growing in my belly – I can't wait to meet you.

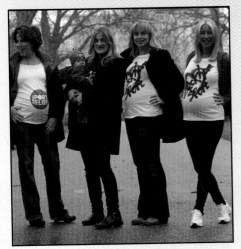

The Bumps and Babies Mile – despite it being freezing cold and pouring with rain, nothing could stop us from raising money for Sport Relief.

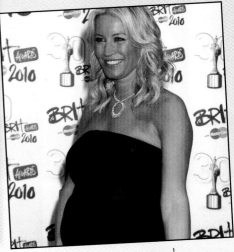

Baby on board at the Brit Awards, a first for me not to take advantage of the hospitality bar.

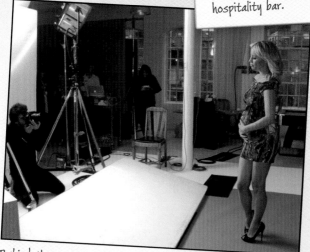

Behind the scenes at a photo shoot for a magazine. Don't be fooled by the glamorous heels, they stayed on for all of five minutes.

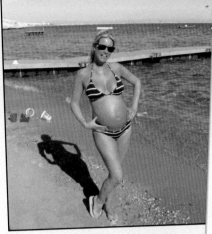

It was nice to feel the warm sun on my bump – well, vitamin D is good for the baby.

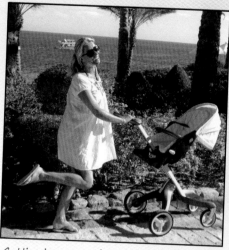

Getting in some early practice with a friend's pram.

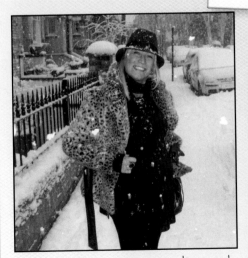

Despite the snow, I took care and ventured out. The fresh air did me the world of good.

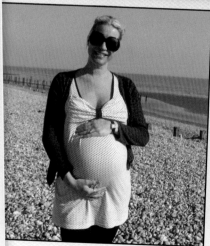

Camber Sands, not far from where we live. Looking forward to paddling in the sea with my daughter.

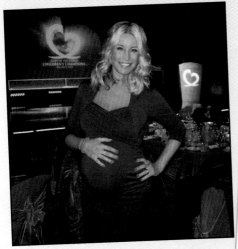

Proudly sporting a dress from my own maternity range at an award ceremony.

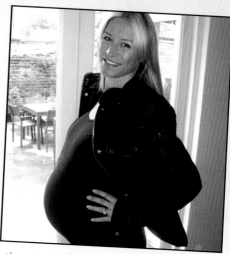

About to head to the hospital, feeling excited and relaxed.

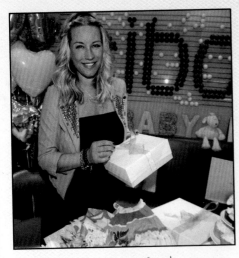

Spoilt rotten by my lovely friends at my baby shower.

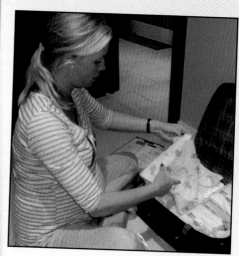

Re-packing my hospital bag for the hundredth time.

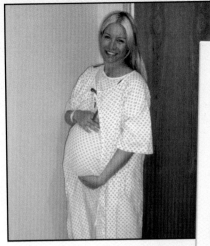

Working the hospital gown.

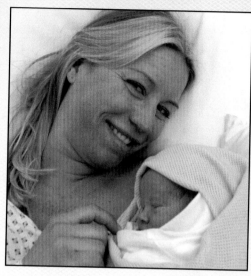

Teapot is finally here. I'm a mum and deliriously happy.

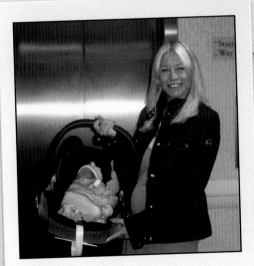

Taking our bundle of joy home.

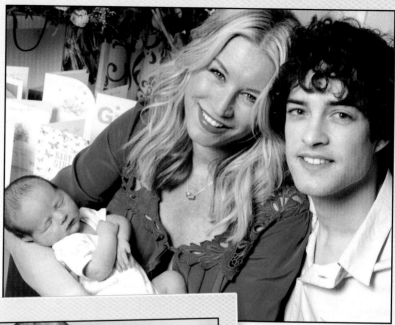

The Meads – our first
family portrait.

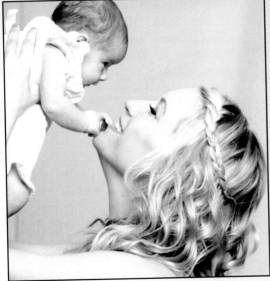

My girl. You're just too good to be true,
can't take my eyes off you.

Eating to sleep well in pregnancy

As Denise mentions this month, as you come into mid-pregnancy, insomnia can become a real problem due to your increased size and the various aches and pains your body will be feeling (not to mention the odd hefty kick from the baby as it gets bigger!). You will also be getting up in the night more often to pee, which can disturb sleep patterns. It's normal, therefore, to feel tired during pregnancy, though it is important to check with your GP if you are suffering from extreme fatigue, as you may need a blood test to determine your iron status. If you are lacking in this vital mineral, you will need to follow your doctor's advice in regard to supplements. Chapter One tells you more about foods that are good for iron.

If all is well on the iron front, then there are some other things you can do to help you to sleep well at night. Although research in the area of how food and drink affects sleep is not terribly conclusive (with the exception of caffeine and alcohol), there is much anecdotal evidence that some eating habits do seem to promote insomnia and are probably worth avoiding, while some appear to help you to nod off. If you are having trouble sleeping, take a look at this twenty-point sleep-promoting checklist:

AVOID...

* **Coffee.** This contains caffeine, a bitter substance that in coffee beans paralyses feasting insects and, in humans, stimulates our central nervous system, making us alert and awake. Some people take just two to three hours to metabolise caffeine in a cup of coffee, others up to eight hours. You may need to stop drinking coffee from early afternoon to aid a good night's sleep. Remember, pregnant women should be having no more than 200 mg of caffeine a day and one mug of coffee contains at least 100 mg.

* **Tea.** While a small 150 ml cup of coffee (the size of an individual yoghurt pot) can provide up to 115 mg of caffeine, a similar-size cup of tea averages only around 40 mg (although it can reach more like 60–70 mg when brewed for a long time). So it is certainly a better choice than coffee, but you still need to watch your overall intake. Caffeine in green and white teas range from 14 mg to 61 mg per mug, while decaffeinated teas can provide up to 12 mg per mug – so even decaff teas can disrupt sleep if you have too many.

* **Cola and energy drinks.** Expect to consume around 40 mg of caffeine in regular and diet colas and up to 150 mg in energy drinks. Avoid especially in the evenings if trying to repair poor sleep patterns.

* **Cold remedies and painkillers.** Check the small print of cold remedies and painkillers. Some have added caffeine that can provide up to 60 mg in a couple of tablets. Only take on the advice of your GP.

* **Dark chocolate.** A 100 g bar of dark chocolate can provide 80 mg of caffeine, along with other potentially stimulating compounds. Stick with a small section of dark chocolate or switch to milk chocolate, with 40 mg of caffeine per 100 g.

* **Alcohol.** The advice while pregnant and when trying to fall pregnant is to avoid drinking alcohol. Even though alcohol can help you to fall asleep, it then disrupts the really beneficial 'restorative' sleep later in the night, so even if you were considering a small nightcap as a last resort to nod off, it wouldn't help a good night's sleep anyway.

* **Fast foods.** High in calories, regular fast food can lead to weight gain around the middle and chest. This can trigger sleep apnoea, a problem with breathing that causes you to wake regularly during the night. Being tired on waking can make you crave more food and reinforce a cycle of over-eating.

* **Late-night food.** Eating last thing at night can disrupt sleep patterns, especially fast food like pizzas, kebabs, burgers and fries that sit heavily on the stomach. Try to leave around two hours between your last meal and bedtime.

* **Biscuits and puddings.** Some experts recommend avoiding sugar-rich foods before bedtime on the basis that excess sugar raises blood glucose, which can make you more alert. This is therefore another good reason to resist the biscuit tin while watching television, however strong the urge. Try a beautifully fresh, tasty and vibrant-looking fruit salad with fromage frais instead.

* **Cheese.** People often say that cheese 'keeps them awake'. Little scientific evidence supports its sleep-depriving properties directly, although some believe its high fat content means it sits heavily in the stomach, causing indigestion and restlessness especially in later pregnancy.

* **Malted drinks and hot chocolate.** These drinks can give you the equivalent of around four teaspoons of sugar per cup (before you add any extra of your own) and so, somewhat counter-intuitively, these two beverages may be worth avoiding in your quest for peaceful slumber.

* **Guarana drinks.** Guarana, which comes from the berries of a South America plant, contains guaranine, a compound with similar characteristics to caffeine. It is known to make you jittery and delay sleeping. You will find around 30 mg of guaranine in a typical guarana drink.

* **Ginger.** Herbalists refer to ginger as a 'stimulating' herb, so it may well be worth avoiding ginger tea infusions prior to bedtime. You should be careful about how much ginger you have in your diet anyway when pregnant; see Chapter Three.

* **Ginseng.** If anyone suggests taking the herb ginseng to boost your energy, don't do it. You shouldn't have it while pregnant and high doses of it have been associated with nervousness and insomnia.

* **Coffee ice cream.** Go easy on luxury ice creams with 'coffee' in the name; they can contain up to 58 mg of caffeine per serving. They are fatty and sugary and are therefore worth avoiding anyway.

DO EAT...

* **Regularly.** Sleep experts tell us that people who eat at regular intervals throughout the day usually have more regular sleep habits.

* **Carbs.** A carbohydrate-rich dinner may also help you to relax and sleep well. Carbohydrates are said to help in the production of the feel-good, de-stressing brain chemical, serotonin. Baked potatoes, pasta, rice and noodles all fit the bill.

* **Turkey.** Turkey, like milk, contains the amino acid tryptophan, which has been dubbed a 'natural sleep inducer'. No good clinical research backs up these claims, but if you fancy a turkey sandwich for dinner, the carbohydrate in the bread may have similarly soporific effects as rice and pasta.

DRINK...

* **Chamomile tea.** An old remedy, but an effective one. Chamomile contains plant compounds that have similar effects on areas of brains as anti-anxiety drugs, helping us to relax and de-stress.

* **Hot milk.** Milk contains the protein building block tryptophan, an amino acid said to enhance sleep, although one cup probably does not contain enough to have a sedative effect. Its soothing benefits may simply be psychological, but if it works for you, it works.

A word on dreams

If, like Denise mentioned in the previous chapter, you have been suffering from disturbing dreams during your pregnancy, be assured they are common and normal, and in no way a portent of things to come. It is hardly surprising that with the huge life change you are about to experience, your subconscious is working overtime to process your thoughts and fears. Throw pregnancy hormones and frequent night waking into the mix (which means you are more likely to remember your dreams), and you have a recipe for some weird and wonderful night-time visions. Laugh them off and try not to dwell on any upsetting ones.

Chapter Eight

New Year, New Fear
Month Six of Pregnancy

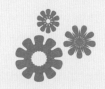

What's going on in your body?

By Week Twenty-two, your baby will be around 27 cm long (this is measured from head to foot from this point onwards, hence the big jump since the previous month). It should now be moving around vigorously and you may feel it respond to touch or a loud noise nearby. You can hear its heartbeat through a stethoscope (your partner may even be able to hear it by putting an ear to your bump). As well as the lanugo, your baby is now also covered in a white, greasy substance called 'vernix', which protects the baby's skin (this mostly disappears before birth). It will be swallowing small amounts of the amniotic fluid inside your womb and passing tiny amounts of urine back into it. At around Week Twenty-six, your baby's eyelids will open for the first time. The eyes are almost always blue or dark blue – most babies are born with blue eyes, only changing to their 'true' colour a few weeks after birth.

Week Twenty-four is another important milestone for you as this is the point at which a baby is 'viable', meaning it has a chance of survival if it is born prematurely. Every week your pregnancy continues from now on increases its odds dramatically.

My Diary

With some spare time to relax in early January I headed to our cottage in Kent. It was the perfect opportunity to catch up on the pregnancy magazines I'd been too busy to read over Christmas and to get my head around the ever-nearing birth. Unfortunately the seclusion also gave me time to dwell on some of the horror stories I had been told since announcing my pregnancy. Everyone had a friend of a friend who had haemorrhaged or had torn really badly during labour. There was someone who didn't even realise she was in labour until she was eight centimetres dilated and another whose waters broke at a train station. One thing's for sure, I would be mortified if my waters broke while I was out in public. (That said, I had heard that if it happens when you're shopping in Harrods they send you a huge hamper full of goodies, which doesn't sound too bad.)

I'd also heard that it's common to empty your bowels during labour so I made the decision to speak to Lee and inform him of the benefits of remaining up at the 'head end'.

With my fears either addressed or pushed to the back of my mind, I was thrilled to receive a letter from the Portland Hospital inviting me to take a look around. It would be the perfect opportunity to familiarise myself with the labour ward and hopefully ensure I was calmer when the day arrived. I know it seems a cliché because lots of people in the public eye have their babies at the Portland in London, but I have been a patient there for my gynaecology check-ups for years so I was already comfortable with the place.

During the tour I visited the labour ward, the private rooms and the operating theatre. One thing that startled me was the amount of equipment everywhere, but I felt much better once one of the midwives had talked me through what everything did. The staff were so lovely and told me they'd see me very soon, so I left feeling really excited. On my way out I bumped into a couple in the lift; the mum-to-be was on a bed while her partner stood next to her wearing a hospital gown. They looked so nervous I wanted to give them both a hug and say, 'It'll be OK, you'll get to meet your baby soon,' but I managed to restrain myself and left them to it. I did speak to a young girl outside who was cautiously loading her newborn baby into the back of a car. I went over to her and congratulated her, and she thanked me before telling me she'd had an emergency Caesarean after complications, but both she and her baby were healthy, which was the main thing. I couldn't help but daydream about how it would feel to be putting Teapot in the back of the car and taking her home to my flat in Hampstead for the first time.

My experiences that day made me view the hospital so differently to how I had seen it before. I'd been going there for years but hadn't thought of it as somewhere where so much life begins. I'd now witnessed it as the magical place it was, where in roughly twelve weeks my life would change forever.

As D-Day approached, it seemed like the perfect time to learn more about what I could expect in labour. With Lee away, I didn't really fancy attending NCT (National Childbirth Trust) classes on my own so I called a midwife who came highly recommended by a mate. Rebecca came and gave me a private session at my flat where we covered everything from how I'd know I was in labour (back pains, pains in my stomach which feel like period pains, feeling like I needed to go for a number two) to breathing through the contractions (or surges as she liked to call them). By the time we were done I felt a lot more confident about the whole chain of events and was certain that I wanted to opt for an epidural as soon as possible when the time came. Call me a cop-out but I hate the thought of being in pain – even the thought of visiting the dentist brings me out in a cold sweat – and knowing the way I am about it, I didn't want to have such a life-changing experience marred by something that can actually be avoided.

Another important part of my preparation was to meet up with a maternity nurse who came highly recommended by a friend. A maternity nurse is someone who moves into your home and helps to look after the baby for the first few weeks. I wasn't sure whether I needed or would want so much help but I was keen to return to work quite soon after having Teapot. The nurse was lovely and she talked me through the benefits of having a routine for the baby, but I decided it would be best for us to find our own way. The whole idea of having a routine scared me; call me naïve but I didn't think it worked that way. I just thought babies knew when to sleep and when to be awake. I began reading various books that covered everything from very strict regimes involving precise timing and blackout blinds, to more flexible routines that I personally thought would suit Lee and I much more.

Like most pregnant women, my eagerness to nest and get everything ready for our new arrival had kicked in really early, but I was paranoid something might happen if I got too ahead of myself so had deliberately held back from choosing any nursery furniture for fear of jinxing the pregnancy. Having visited the hospital, the time now felt right, so I started the exciting task of kitting out the nursery. First stop: Mamas and Papas, to look for a cot, and I soon realised I'd underestimated how many things you need to take into consideration. One friend had advised me to get a cot bed because it would last for years, while another told me her baby found the transition from a Moses basket to a cot bed very difficult because it was so big. After what felt like hours of quizzing a helpful assistant (bless her, I think she was glad to see the back of me), looking at every one of the cots and cot beds in the shop and weighing up the pros and cons, I decided on the perfect cot. It felt so good and a little emotional as I placed my order.

Next on my list was Mothercare, to stock up on all of the essentials. Another friendly assistant very kindly walked me around the shop, pointing out all the things I'd need. I couldn't believe how much there was to buy, everything from breast pads to sanitary towels – and not just a few, but literally bundles of each. Perineal oil was something I'd never even heard of before but I now know it's a special oil you massage down below to make the skin more supple and to reduce the chances of the skin tearing during the birth. I ended up at the checkout with baskets full of stuff. I was definitely going to need to clear out a few more cupboards to accommodate it all (more shoes relegated to storage then). The assistant also suggested I popped to Primark over the road to invest in some cheap big knickers and leggings for when I came out of hospital. Now that's the kind of advice you can't find in any pregnancy book. Well, not until now anyway!

The next thing I needed was a car seat, something I'd been advised to get fairly early on because hospitals won't actually allow you to take your baby home unless you have one fitted in your car. My new second home, the fourth floor of John Lewis, seemed the best place for a road test. As we all know, London's black cab drivers are famous for having something to say about everything, but the cabbie who took me to Oxford Street had a really in-depth knowledge about car seats and recommended the Isofix system, which sounded more like a sports drink than something I'd need for my baby. Sure enough, he was right and the guys at John Lewis showed me how having an Isofix fitted into the car makes it so much easier to put the baby seat in and out every time.

As the nursery furniture and parcels started to arrive at my door I was so thrilled, more so than if I'd received a delivery from Topshop which was usually enough to induce a flurry of excitement. Each time something new arrived I'd unwrap it and test it to make sure I knew how it worked. This is another thing I'd highly recommend, not only so you can get excited about your new purchase but also to ensure that everything is in working order before your baby arrives. Discovering the steriliser you've bought is faulty at the last minute would be a nightmare, especially if the twenty-eight day exchange policy has expired. Let's face it, none of us likes to waste money.

By now I was feeling very heavy and by the end of the day my back and feet would be killing me. If I accidentally dropped something on the floor I would struggle to pick it up. That was until a genius friend came up with the idea of using BBQ tongs, which I have to admit I started using all the time around the flat. Not so useful though when I was out and about: imagine the stares I would have got on Hampstead High Street pulling out my tongs to reclaim my travel card.

So far throughout my pregnancy I'd been careful to stick to Amanda's healthy eating plan, with the odd exception of a slice of cake or two and my regular hot chocolates, but now my self control was slowly going out of the window. I think it was psychological, as the closer I got to the end of my pregnancy the more I let myself go. I'd started opting for chips as a side order whenever I ate out and was buying more biscuits and snacks for the kitchen cupboard. Determined not to pile on any extra pounds I didn't need, I came up with a cunning plan to help me stick to being healthy. Every January without fail I hit the Sales, so I decided to pick up a few last-minute bargains as an incentive, to motivate me to get back into shape once Teapot had arrived. First stop was Selfridges, where I had a good rummage through the rails and picked up a gorgeous little dress and jacket. As I stood in front of the mirror with the jacket on, unable to zip it up, I found myself having one of those dream-sequence moments like in the movies where everything goes blurry for a couple of seconds and you then reappear as the new you. In my mind's eye I was slim and healthy and the outfit looked fantastic, but somehow I don't think the shop assistant shared my vision as she threw me a bemused look as if to say, 'You have *got* to be kidding me.'

Despite feeling huge and constantly tired, I decided to take the advice of a couple of my mates who already have children and get out as much as possible before I was tied to the house. I set about replying to a pile of invites that had accumulated on the mantelpiece. The next few weeks were now set to be busy with fashion shows, parties and award ceremonies.

On my first night out I was over the moon to be reunited with my fellow Kilimanjaro trekkers, most of whom I hadn't seen since the trek. It was the first time many had seen me pregnant and everyone was so thrilled for me. The celebration at the luxurious five-star Mandarin Oriental Hotel in London's Knightsbridge was to mark the tenth wedding anniversary of Gary Barlow and his wife, Dawn. The evening began with a montage of videos and pictures of the happy couple, including early pictures of when Gary and Dawn first got together, Dawn when she was heavily pregnant, and then with their children on family holidays. The first thing that struck me was that Gary had taken his family to some fabulous places. The pressure is on Lee (not that I'm high maintenance)! The second thing I noticed about all of the pictures was just how happy everyone looked and what great fun they seemed to be having, splashing around in the sea and building sandcastles. I was filled with a sense of pleasure and excitement at the thought of starting on the same road with Lee, and began imagining all the family holidays that lay ahead for us.

Up until now, my holidays had only ever consisted of me covering myself in suncream, hitting the beach for hours and only moving to grab a cocktail. In fact I remember my fabulous holiday with David Walliams on the island of Kurumba in the Maldives – he was training for his Comic Relief swim at the time so was always in the sea swimming back and forth for hours on end; it was exhausting to watch. Sporadically I'd leave my spot to sit in the shallow part of the sea for a minute or so before returning to my lounger. On one occasion when David finally returned from his mammoth workout he surprised me by asking, 'Are you popping into the sea for a wee?' Damn, I thought I was being super-discreet but the guilt was written all over my face. Needless to say, he took the pee (excuse the pun) for the rest of our stay. To make matters worse my beach villa was a mere stone's throw away from where I was lazing.

Back to the party, and after dinner Gary took up his role as a bingo caller with guests receiving their own lucky card. There were fabulous prizes to be won, with one in particular catching my eye. I had an overwhelming feeling I was going to win it, so as the first number was called I turned to Fearne Cotton who was my date for the evening and told her the prize was mine. As Gary called the numbers I was busy crossing them off and before I knew it I was shouting, 'House!' I'd won a day of treatments at the award-winning Mandarin Oriental Spa. Later that evening I bumped into Dawn and she told me how pleased she was that I'd won, especially as the spa does a fabulous pregnancy massage, one that she had treated herself to the last time she was pregnant. She went on to explain how strange it was that I had bagged that particular prize, especially as she'd mentioned to Gary how great it would be for me to win. It was meant to be. I was going to indulge in a day of pure bliss before Teapot arrived.

Now for the Experts...

Preparing your body for birth

By the sixth month of your pregnancy, as Denise found, you will start to look ahead more seriously and think about the impending birth. It's a good idea to start attending antenatal classes if you haven't already, so you are mentally and physically prepared for what is to come. Ask your doctor or midwife for details of local classes, or you can even buy DVDs that guide you through the process and teach you the relaxation and breathing techniques you will need on the big day. Remember, the more preparation for labour that you do in advance, the less scared you will feel when it starts happening for real.

You can also start doing some simple exercises at home that help to strengthen the muscle groups that you'll be using when you give birth. You can start these any time from your first trimester, ideally two or three times a week. In addition, try to keep up your general fitness routine as outlined earlier, as this will improve your overall energy levels, strength and endurance, all of which will also help you during labour.

Exercises to help you prepare for labour

Seated Curl

1 Sit on the floor with plenty of cushions behind your back for support. Bend your legs up, keeping your knees shoulder-width apart, so you are leaning back in a semi-reclined position. Place your hands on your thighs.

2 Breathe in, and gently tilt your pelvis upwards so your upper body curls into a C-shape. Pull your stomach muscles in towards your spine while you relax your pelvic floor muscles, and keep your chin up.

3 Hold this position for five seconds while you slowly exhale, then relax. Take two deep breaths in between each set. Repeat two or three times. This exercise strengthens the abdominal muscles you will be using when you're pushing your baby out.

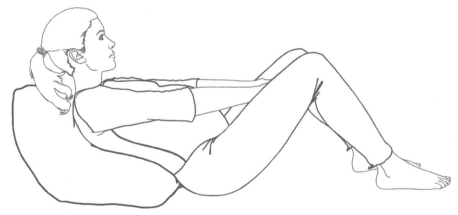

Lower Back Stretch

1 Get down on your hands and knees, with your knees under your hips and hands under your shoulders, and your head and neck in line with your spine.

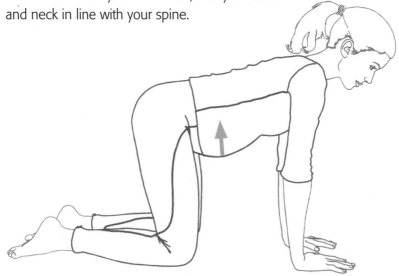

2 Breathe in deeply, then gently breathe out, tightening your stomach muscles as you do so and imagining you are pulling your baby in towards your spine.

3 Relax for a few seconds, but don't let your stomach sag or back arch. Aim for two sets of eight to ten repetitions. This is similar to the Arched Cat stretch on page 69, so it's a great back pain reliever as well as helping to strengthen your abdominal muscles.

Supported Squat

1 Stand next to a table or chair with your feet slightly wider than hip-width apart, toes in line with your knees.
2 Holding on with one hand for support, squat down slowly, pushing your weight down through your heels and contracting your stomach muscles. Keep your chest lifted and shoulders relaxed.
3 Return to a standing position and repeat ten times. This exercise strengthens your thighs and helps open up your pelvis.

Butterfly Stretch

1 Sit on the floor with your back supported against a wall and the soles of your feet touching each other.

2 Pull your feet in towards you, then gently use your elbows to press your knees down. Hold this position as long as you're comfortable but remember not to overstretch. This will help to open up your pelvis and loosen your hip joints in preparation for birth, as well as improve your posture and ease tension in your lower back.

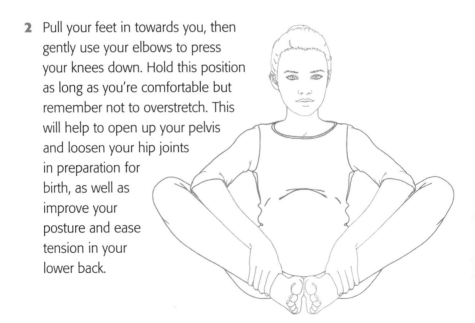

Tricep Curl

1 On a mat or carpeted floor, kneel on your left knee beside a chair, keeping your right foot forward and flat on the floor. Keep your knees at right angles, with your left knee directly under your hip and your right directly over your heel.

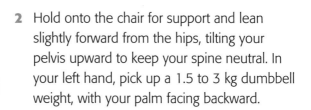

2 Hold onto the chair for support and lean slightly forward from the hips, tilting your pelvis upward to keep your spine neutral. In your left hand, pick up a 1.5 to 3 kg dumbbell weight, with your palm facing backward.

3 Bend your left elbow up and back while pulling your shoulder blades together, bringing it far enough back to feel a stretch in your chest muscles but without rotating your upper body.

4 Slowly return to the starting position. Do eight to ten reps with the left arm, then switch arms, aiming for two sets on each side. This exercise strengthens your triceps, upper back and shoulder muscles, which will help you to keep your chest open during labour, making breathing easier.

> **Remember:** *keep up your pelvic floor exercises as described on page 51. These are vital for strengthening your PC muscles and teaching you to relax them during the pushing phase of labour.*

Healthy Snacking in pregnancy

Denise mentioned this month that, however hard she tried, by now she was finding it really difficult to stick with healthy eating and was more and more tempted to give in to the urge for biscuits and crisps.

Any pregnant woman knows this feeling. There is something about being so much larger than you are used to being that makes you feel that you may as well indulge. After all, no one will really notice, and few extra pounds put on here and there won't hurt.

The truth is, a few pounds may not hurt you directly and if you try really hard, you can probably get them off again after the birth. However, the best way of staying on track as much as possible is to refer to the research mentioned in Chapter Three, which showed that the danger of eating high-fat food is that it may affect your baby's long-term future health as well as contributing to your own excessive weight gain in the short term, increasing your child's risk of obesity and raised cholesterol in later life.

So while there will be times when you absolutely can not resist, if you try to think about the effects the food you are about to eat will have on your growing baby, it may just give you the extra resolve you need.

However, while you should try to resist the things that may potentially harm your growing baby, it is worth being realistic and acknowledging that a mum in the latter stages of pregnancy does need about 200–300 extra calories per day. So if you know which snacks are the least likely to dramatically raise your blood sugar and fat levels, then you can still build treats into your day as long as the rest of your diet is well balanced.

The lists below provide a guide to healthy snacks that fulfil your desire for a bit of indulgence, while also taking care of your baby's health. As well as being just 100 calories each, these snacks raise blood sugar levels in your (and therefore your baby's) body fairly gently. They are either low in fat or – if slightly higher in fat – contribute mostly 'good' fats that do not raise bad cholesterol.

Filling snacks

These snacks have the advantage of filling you up, but adding other useful nutrients too.

- Handful of almonds
- Slice of toast with peanut butter
- A slice of malt loaf
- Toasted crumpet with a thin slice of half-fat Cheddar
- Slice of toast with a tablespoon of hummus

'Naughty but not' snacks

Surprisingly, ice cream, in small servings, does not make blood sugar levels shoot up. If you have it with fruit, it helps to keep levels more stable.

- A slice of ice cream roll (50 g)
- One scoop of ice cream (55 g)
- Baked apple with a tablespoon of fruit yoghurt
- Six slices of peaches canned in natural juice with a small meringue and a heaped teaspoon of fromage frais
- Creamy pineapple smoothie (blend 100 ml of skimmed milk with a slice of pineapple canned in natural juice and a tablespoon of 0% fat Greek yoghurt)

Bone-building snacks

These snacks have the advantage of giving you the mineral calcium as well as being tasty and satisfying.

- 'Tall' decaffeinated cappuccino from a coffee shop or a homemade one with 170 ml skimmed milk and a good sprinkling of chocolate
- Small pot of 0% fat Greek yoghurt with a swirl of honey
- Big bowl of your favourite berries with a blob of low-fat fruit fromage frais
- Individual crème caramel (100 g)
- Ready-made pot of low-fat rice pudding (100 g)

Comfort snacks

If you need a bit of comfort food, then try tucking into one of these options. Ones marked with an asterisk contain the least salt.

- 220 ml mug of hot canned cream of tomato soup
- 1 bag of baked crisps
- Two crispbreads with a thin slice of reduced-fat Cheddar and some sliced cucumber
- A chicken drumstick (minus skin) and a few cherry tomatoes*
- An oatcake topped with ricotta cheese and a crunchy carrot or celery stick*
- 100 g of tzatziki (or low-fat yoghurt-style dip) with a raw carrot cut into chunks or batons*
- 1 tablespoon of low-fat cream cheese, two breadsticks and a chunk of cucumber*

Chocolate snacks

If you really need a chocolate snack then portion control is probably your best option. So buy a small bar and eat it slowly. The best way to avoid going back for more is to never keep chocolate in your house, so you only go out and get some when the urge is overwhelming. Remember that 50 g of dark chocolate has up to 40 mg of caffeine in it, which is one fifth of your daily maximum intake, while the same serving of milk chocolate has around 10 mg of caffeine.

Real chocolate is better than bars with toffee and other sweet additions because the latter raise blood sugar more than chocolate on its own.

Dairy Milk Freddo *95 calories, 5.4 g fat per 18 g bar*
The Freddo bar comes in at pole position simply because of its serving size. With just 18 g of chocolate it is perfect portion control, giving milk chocolate lovers a little bit of what they fancy, without being tempted to wolf down a big bar.

Ador Dark Chocolate or **Green & Black's Dark Chocolate** *179 calories, 16 g fat per 35 g bar*
This chocolate again represents good portion control for dark chocolate lovers. Research shows that eating dark chocolate that is brittle and quite hard to digest helps to keep you feeling full for longer. The research showed that a small serving of dark chocolate reduced calorie intake at a subsequent meal by up to eighteen per cent. Ador has the added advantage of containing some pine nut oil fatty acids, which are believed to add to this hunger-beating effect.

Kit Kat *107 calories, 5.4 g fat per 21 g bar (two fingers)*
A two-finger Kit Kat has always been a pretty good option for a lowish calorie chocolate splurge. There is no need to exercise portion control because if you buy the two-finger pack, you can eat the lot for just 107 calories. And because much of the product is biscuit, the fat and saturated fat are implicitly pretty low.

Other calorie-controlled chocolate bars include the **Twix Fino**, with 94 calories per finger, a 26 g **Curly Wurly** bar containing 115 calories, one **Flight** bar from a 45 g twin pack, which contains 97 calories, or half a small 37 g bag of **Maltesers** with 93 calories.

Chapter Nine

Outen About
Month Seven of Pregnancy

What's going on in your body?

Congratulations, you are now in your third and final trimester! Your baby should now measure around 36 cm from head to foot and weigh around 1 kg (the same as a bag of sugar) – though it may feel like much more than that when you take into account the weight of the placenta, amniotic fluid and extra blood that's coursing round your system.

Your baby is gradually becoming less wrinkled as he lays down more fat stores under his skin. Now his eyes are open, he can see bright lights through your skin (assuming you've taken your top off!). From around Week Twenty-eight, a further period of brain development begins: the amount of brain tissue increases and grooves and channels start to appear on its previously smooth surface.

By the end of the month, your baby is likely to be moving less in the womb. This is nothing to worry about: it's simply becoming a bit of a tight squeeze in there. However, if you don't feel your baby move for a whole day, call your midwife just to check everything is OK.

As for you, your growing uterus may leave you short of breath, and your skin may feel tight and itchy. If you haven't already suffered from the joys of swollen feet or ankles, constipation, piles, gum disease or urinary tract infections, this might be when it starts to happen. Oh, the glamour of pregnancy! On the plus side, your skin and hair should still be looking fabulous – and anyway, your baby won't care what you look like when you meet him…

My Diary

The Brit Awards is always one of my favourite dates in my social calendar and it just so happened to be the first of my ambitious number of RSVPs for the month. I've been attending the ceremony for as long as I can remember and it's always a pretty raucous night out, but this year was obviously going to be more subdued and tamer than I'm used to, so it would be interesting to see things from a teetotal perspective.

I felt mixed emotions on the red carpet – a little rebellious just being there while sporting a full-on bump, but I was also slightly apprehensive as it was the first big night out I'd had in a while. I'd opted for a stylish floor-length black dress that showed off my bump nicely, and heels that felt comfy at the start of the evening but would no doubt become increasingly harder to walk in as the night progressed. The photographers flashed away, all with wide-angled lenses I'm sure. It's funny to think that a few years ago they'd have been banking on bagging a shot of me looking slightly worse for wear later on in the evening and now they'd be more likely to catch me adjusting my big granny knickers or smuggling a doggie bag into my handbag for the journey home.

Once inside I headed straight to the loo only to find a queue half a mile long, which isn't the most welcome sight when you're heavily pregnant and just want to sit down. Luckily an attendant spotted me joining the back of the huge line and came to my rescue, ushering me into the disabled toilet. I only needed to retouch my lip-gloss and powder my nose, but hey, if you can't skip a queue or two when you're pregnant then when can you? In fact, while I'm on the subject of relieving oneself when pregnant, I'd been dying to test the law that apparently states a policeman has to give up his helmet to a pregnant lady if she's caught short. Maybe I could muster up the courage to give it a go before Teapot arrived?

Back at the Brits, my mate Sam and I took our places for dinner, which was already much more civilised than any Brits experience I'd had in the past. A far cry from 1997 when my *Big Breakfast* sidekick Johnny Vaughn and I gave it large after receiving the OK from our boss to come in tired the following morning to present the show. I thought I was so cool back then in my skin-tight blue rubber dress complementing my bright orange tan and peroxide blonde hair, which was pulled back in the tightest of ponytails. I remember sitting backstage in the exclusive artists' bar and loving every minute, drinking JD and Coke while smoking away like a trouper. That outing was when Johnny and I first realised just how popular the *Big Breakfast* show had become, because so many people came up to us throughout the evening to tell us they watched every morning and how brilliant they thought it was. From what I can remember of the following morning, the show went surprisingly well considering we were still drinking at 2 a.m. and rehearsals began just a couple of hours later. Somehow it feels like a different lifetime and yet I can remember it like it was yesterday. All of my stamina in '97 was used to stay awake and party hard but now I needed every ounce of energy just to stay on my feet and carry my huge bump around.

Despite feeling on the large side I was still determined to enjoy the night by having a little boogie, and I was first up when Lady Gaga took to the stage. It was amazing; as soon as she started singing 'Poker Face', Teapot began to move around like she was dancing along too. First an elbow then a foot came poking out – there was definitely a little routine coming together inside my belly. I swear she recognised the song from when it was on a loop constantly in the car and was appreciating the extra bass that was vibrating around the arena from the live performance. It was reassuring to think that she already had great taste in music.

The night was a good opportunity to catch up with some friends: Fearne, Robbie and Ronan to name a few. There were also plenty of journalists keen to catch up with me, and as you'd expect, my pregnancy, cravings and relationship with Lee were hot topics of conversation. I'd been happily chatting away to each reporter until a journalist from the *Daily Mail* asked me how I felt about not being part of the new BBC show *Over the Rainbow*. Her question took me by surprise and I had to rack my brain for something to say. Despite my best efforts to remain cheerful it put a real damper on the rest of my evening.

In spite of having much-sought-after tickets for all the coolest after-parties I decided to call it a night as Take That took to the stage for the big finale. My feet were killing me and my mood was subdued, so I headed home for a relatively early night. As soon as I got through my front door I took my shoes off to survey the damage and I had clearly pushed the glamour to the limit. Everything from my knees downwards was swollen to the point where I had canckles (ankles and calves merged as one) and my feet resembled plates of meat. I had luncheon feet! There was nothing for it: my relationship with high heels was now on hold until after Teapot was born.

The following morning I woke to a barrage of messages, with everyone wanting to know my feelings on being ousted from the new show. The headlines read, 'Denise Van Outen Axed from Show Due to Pregnancy.' I took some time to think and chatted to Lee over breakfast before deciding there was nothing for me to say. Obviously I was hugely disappointed but I wasn't going to wallow in it and let it affect my pregnancy any more than it already had. It's funny because it was as if Teapot knew when I was getting stressed out or upset, as she'd give me a little kick to let me know she was there.

With my heels safely packed away, it was time to get my trainers on for my next engagement. Having seen first-hand where the money raised for Sport Relief goes I had been extremely keen to organise another charity event, especially as I was unable to take part in the 1,000-mile cycle ride from Land's End to John O'Groats. So I recruited five pregnant celebrity mums-to-be to join me in the first Sports Relief 'Bumps And Babies Mile', to encourage people to sign up for the Sport Relief mile and do their bit for charity. My fellow mum-to-be walkers included newsreader Natasha Kaplinsky, Joe Cole's wife Carly Zucker and actress Kim Medcalf, and we had a whale of a time comparing notes on everything from tiredness, aches and pains to weird cravings. I'm sure there were more than a few eyebrows raised as we waddled our way around London's Battersea Park in our big t-shirts and leggings, but we were blissfully unaware in our bubble of baby loveliness. Towards the end I was thankful that I had kept up my training with Nicki as I found it relatively easy compared to some of the other girls who were beginning to get out of breath and struggle.

The next big outing for Teapot and I was a fashion show to raise money to help survivors of the horrific Haiti earthquake. The event, which took place during London Fashion Week, was organised by supermodel Naomi Cambell and was extremely star-studded, as she had called on a host of her celebrity friends to walk the catwalk. I arrived to be greeted with a huge hug from Naomi who couldn't thank me enough for making the effort to join her. Backstage was buzzing as Dame Shirley Bassey, Geri Halliwell, Kimberley Walsh and Alexandra Burke were getting preened and pampered in preparation for hitting the runway. I was thrilled to be going on the same catwalk as so many fabulous people but my excitement went into overdrive when I spotted Kate Moss, whom I've admired for a very long time. A mutual friend could see my excitement so led me over to say hello. It was clear she was already a little bit merry and didn't seem to want to chat. I was disappointed. Naomi, on the other hand, couldn't have been nicer, checking I was OK for water and making me feel part of the event. She also told me she was gutted that I wouldn't be on *Over the Rainbow* as she was a really big fan of the previous shows and thought I was an important part of the panel. It was really lovely of her to say that to me and lifted my mood even more for the evening. Who knew I had a supermodel fan?

My catwalk partner-in-crime for the night was Amanda Holden, who was absolutely brilliant and did a great job of stabilising me as I did my best impression of a catwalk model in super-high heels with a centre of gravity close to that of an elephant. After having my hair and make-up done professionally and donning a stunning cream dress, I felt better than I had for a few weeks, although slightly nervous. I'd only ever walked the catwalk once before at a Vivienne Westwood show years ago, but on that occasion I was off balance because of all the champagne I'd drunk to give me Dutch courage.

Once our stint was over, Amanda and I could relax, and I got the opportunity to quiz her on how she feels about being a mum. She told me that having her daughter Lexi was the best thing that has ever happen to her and that motherhood had changed her life in so many positive ways. Every day Lexi makes her laugh by coming out with something cute and unexpected. They make up songs and dance routines together at home and put on private performances, plus she's had the opportunity to relive her own childhood by sitting down with her daughter to watch the old Disney classics. All of these things I couldn't wait to do with my little girl. She also stressed how important it is to not feel guilty about working, and that the key is to make sure that the time you do get to spend with your child is quality time. They were welcome words of wisdom from someone who has experienced first-hand what I had to come. Lastly she assured me that whenever she's had a hard day at work the best feeling in the world is coming home to a huge cuddle and gorgeous smile from someone who loves you unconditionally.

Now for the Experts...

As long as your doctor or midwife has given you the all-clear and you're not officially at risk of delivering a pre-term baby, it's still safe to exercise in the third trimester. However, if you've been doing quite high-impact exercise up to now, you should review your routine and start taking it more gently. Don't lift heavy weights, as your tendons and ligaments are becoming even more stretchy in late pregnancy, so they are at risk of tearing. As ever, listen to your body and stop exercising if you feel any of the symptoms listed on page 50. Call your doctor if you experience vaginal bleeding or leaking of watery fluid, severe headaches, decreased foetal movement, a marked increase in swelling, constant or severe abdominal pain, or more than five contractions an hour (particularly if you are less than thirty-seven weeks pregnant).

Try to keep up your abdominal and back exercises as listed on pages 134–7, as they will help with the postural changes associated with the baby engaging into your pelvis, which will happen in a few weeks. You'll also have to do a lot of lifting once the baby is born, so it's good to anticipate this and strengthen those muscles beforehand.

As mentioned previously, you mustn't lie on your back in late pregnancy, so don't do abdominal crunches lying down. Instead lie on your side or on your hands and knees, and try to bring your navel towards your spine. You can also do standing pelvic tilts against a wall.

Sex (remember that?) is still safe in the third trimester, unless you're at risk for pre-term labour. But as lying on your back is not recommended, experiment with positions where you are on top or you are both lying on your side.

It's usual to feel absolutely huge in this stage of pregnancy, but speak to your doctor or midwife if you feel concerned that you are gaining too much weight. They may be able to reassure you that it's within the 'normal' range, even if you feel like you can hardly fit through a door these days. Remember that exercise can help with these body issues because it will give you a feeling of control over your body, and release some endorphins into the bargain. So although you're not exercising to lose weight at this stage, it's important to stay active.

Finally, make sure you get enough rest. It's hard to sleep at night in this trimester so try to take naps when you can during the day. If that's not possible, then at least give yourself a five-minute break every hour, in which you do some deep breathing exercises and try to relax your body. A quick walk round the block in the fresh air can have a rejuvenating effect if you are struggling to focus.

Suggested regime:

* **Gentle exercise** three times a week for thirty minutes, such as two sessions of walking and one of swimming
  plus
* One weekly pregnancy **pilates** or **yoga** class, or an antenatal **aquacise** class.

Two gentle toning moves you can do in late pregnancy

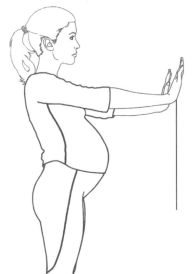

Wall Plié

1 Stand facing a wall, with your feet slightly farther than hip-width apart and your knees turned out. Place your hands on the wall and tilt your pelvis so your tailbone points down.

2 Bend your knees slowly, lowering your torso toward the floor.

3 Then straighten up, pressing your weight through your heels, and repeat. Do one or two sets of ten repetitions, resting one minute between each set.

Wall Push-Up

1 Stand facing a wall as above, with your feet hip-width apart. Place your hands on the wall, keeping your arms straight. Make sure your back is straight and pull your navel in towards your spine.

2 Bend your elbows, bringing your chest towards the wall.

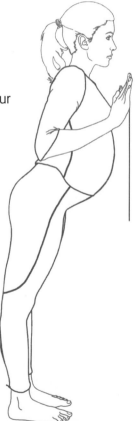

3 Push back and repeat. Do one or two sets of ten reps, resting one minute between each set.

Perineal massage

Daily perineal massage starting from around six weeks before the birth is another good way to prepare your body for labour and delivery. The perineum is the area between the vagina and the rectum, which stretches and thins during labour when the baby's head emerges. Massaging this area regularly helps to make it stretch more easily, reducing the chances of tearing or an episiotomy (a cut to help the baby out) when you give birth. Before starting, wash your hands thoroughly with soap and hot water and make sure your fingernails are trimmed. Sit comfortably with your legs spread apart or stand with one foot up on a chair. Apply some K-Y jelly or massage oil to your thumbs and insert them in your vagina. Press downward toward your rectum, until you feel a gentle stretching and stinging sensation. Try to keep relaxed and continue to massage the lower part of the vaginal passage back and forth, until you become more used to the feeling.

Eating to avoid indigestion and heartburn

The period from about twenty-eight to thirty-six weeks is usually the worst time for experiencing digestive disorders, as your baby is taking up so much room high up in your body. Once your baby drops down into the pelvis (see page 162) at around thirty-six weeks, you'll find your digestive system has a bit more room and you'll be able to eat more again. Until then, you may find you occasionally suffer from discomfort low down in your stomach, especially after a large meal.

As well as indigestion, you may also experience heartburn, which is a burning sensation at the top of your stomach as its acidic contents are brought back into your oesophagus. As usual, it's your pregnancy hormones that are to blame, as they affect the valve at the top of your stomach. Heartburn usually occurs if you eat late at night.

If you suffer from either of these ailments, try the following suggestions:

* Eat **little and often** – five small meals a day rather than three big ones. Don't eat late at night.

* Eat **slowly** and chew your food well before swallowing.

* **Sit up straight** during and after meals, and let your food digest properly before doing any exercise.

* **Avoid** rich, fatty foods, fizzy drinks, coffee, alcohol and spicy foods.

* Use **cushions** to prop you up when you sleep, to help prevent the acidic stomach contents coming back up.

* Wear **loose, comfortable clothing** with no restrictive waistbands.

* You can take some over-the-counter **antacids** but do check with your pharmacist as some aren't safe to use in pregnancy.

Eating to avoid urinary tract infections

Another annoying problem that can crop up more often than usual during pregnancy is a urinary tract infection, either in the bladder or the tube leading from the bladder to the outside of your body. In some cases it can also affect the kidneys and the tubes that lead from the kidneys to the bladder.

Urinary tract infections are usually caused by bacteria called E. Coli (found on our skin, in the large intestines and in our stools), which find their way into our urinary system where they reproduce and cause a lot of discomfort. You might need to go to the loo more often than usual and experience a severe burning pain when you do go.

Once again it is the changes in your hormones while pregnant that make these infections more common, as well as your bladder not emptying properly due to the growing uterus pressing on it.

If you do experience a urinary tract infection, it needs to be treated quickly to prevent further problems like a full-blown kidney infection. See your doctor if you think you might have one.

Nutritional help comes in the form of prevention. Looking after your immune system is important so check the nutritional information in Chapter Two to help get your immunity working optimally.

Next, aim to drink 300 ml of cranberry juice daily. There is good evidence that the super-nutrients in cranberry juice help to stop E. Coli bacteria from sticking to the sides of the urinary tract, so that they slip off and are passed harmlessly out of your body in your urine.

Drinking enough fluid in general is also important. Try hard to take in up to eight glasses of water a day if you can. You can count herbal teas and fruit juices in this total.

Chapter Ten

They Call It Nesting

Month Eight of Pregnancy

What's going on in your body?

After the rapid growth in length during each of the previous months, your baby will only be growing about 1 cm a week from now on. But he will still be concentrating on 'plumping up' and laying down fat stores. So between Week Thirty-one and the birth, your baby will roughly double his weight, whereas he has already reached around eighty per cent of his birth length now. As a result, you will continue to put on weight – even when you think you can't possibly get any bigger – at the rate of about 500 g a week. You may also notice other changes in your body around this time: the veins on your breasts will be more pronounced, there will be darker markings around your nipples, and possibly some leaking of colostrum (the yellow, creamy milk your body produces for your newborn). Your belly button will also turn inside-out as your bump increases in size!

From Week Thirty-two onwards, your baby has an excellent chance of survival if he is born early, as his lungs are much more mature now, though obviously the longer he stays inside you the more he can put on enough weight to regulate his body temperature when he does come out to face the world. By the end of this month, any time from Week Thirty-four, your baby may start to 'engage', that is, settle head-down (with luck) and move into your pelvis ready for birth. You'll know when your baby has engaged because you will feel the baby's head low down in your pelvic floor muscles. You'll also be able to breathe and eat a bit more easily (at last!) as you'll have some more space in your tummy above the baby.

My Diary

There have been so many times over the years when I've decided to do a short detox by giving the red wine a miss for a week or two and it's literally *guaranteed* that an invite to a party or an event that's just too good to miss lands on my doormat and I end up letting my hair down. Well, it happened again. No sooner had I realised that I really couldn't keep up the pace of the last crazy couple of weeks and made a promise to myself to slow down a bit than I received another one of those invites I just couldn't refuse. The handwritten letter was from Sarah Brown, not inviting me to a booze-fuelled party (although I reckon a glass of wine or two with the former PM's wife would be a lot of fun), but instead asking me to join her and a group of other people who contribute to raising awareness and money for cancer charities in the UK. This really was something I couldn't miss out on – my work for breast cancer is very important to me as I lost my Nan to the disease. Apart from that I'd also thoroughly enjoyed my previous visit to 10 Downing Street that had taken place after the Kilimanjaro trek.

As my car drew up outside No. 10 I was of course incredibly excited, but because I was on my own with no Lee by my side I found myself actually quite nervous. This felt like a really grown-up and serious event and that's the kind of thing I'd normally do with my hubby. Thankfully the security guards broke the ice, and as I was going through the usual security checks for Downing Street they were making jokes and having a giggle about what I was trying to smuggle into the party under my dress (my favourite guess was an upturned wok). As I made my way inside I caught a glimpse of Nicola Roberts from Girls Aloud who looked just as nervous as me, so we made a beeline for each other and agreed to spend the rest of the evening together as moral support.

We were in great company that evening among people who show tireless support for the many cancer charities, and the guests also included people who had been affected by some form or other of cancer and had beaten the awful disease. I found it somewhat comforting to be surrounded by such generous and inspirational people when I was about to bring a new life into the world. It made a really pleasant change from watching the news, which always seems filled with stories of doom and gloom, and people you wouldn't want to bump into on a dark night.

Unsurprisingly, it wasn't long before I needed to pay the first of many visits to the ladies', and not wanting to go alone I roped Nicola in to come with me. Now, you'd think that at Downing Street there would be some kind of visitors' loo just off every reception room so that people don't go wandering around. But there isn't, so despite receiving detailed directions to the nearest loo before we set off, we somehow managed to get lost and found ourselves in what seemed to be a never-ending corridor. Taking a fifty–fifty guess we headed to the bottom and opened a door that led to a huge dining room. Like a couple of schoolgirls we had a quick snoop around before Nicola pointed out another more intriguing wooden door leading off it. There was a good chance that if we went any further alarms could go off and laser targets from the guns of special agents would be pointed at us as we entered the very heart of the British government HQ, all of which was quite exciting. But when I saw a camera tracking us around the room I totally lost my bottle. What was I thinking? I was pregnant and should be acting in a much more grown-up manner, besides which my loo trip was become slightly more urgent if I was to avoid making a mess of the floor.

However, while I was keen to keep the carpets of 10 Downing Street in the same pristine condition as when I arrived, Gordon and Sarah Brown had other ideas.

'Wouldn't it be great if you went into labour right here and now?' they joked.

'No way' was my first thought, not without my hospital bag and certainly not in this dress.

'We could see the headlines now,' they continued. 'Den's definitely in Labour.'

I don't get publicly involved in politics at all, but that would have had a certain comedic value for sure. As I mentioned earlier, I've heard that if your waters break in some shops you get presented with gifts varying from a year's supply of nappies in supermarkets to a luxury hamper in Harrods, so what I really wanted to know was what I'd get if it happened in Downing Street? A lifetime's absolution from parking tickets or a guaranteed place in the cabinet for Teapot when she was old enough? Or maybe even free hire of the party rooms at No. 10 for all of Teapot's birthday parties? How cool would that be?

With the end of my pregnancy now in sight my nesting instinct went into overdrive. I'd lived in my flat for over six years and only now was I noticing its many imperfections, from marks on the ceiling to cracks in the woodwork. I was a woman possessed as I marched from room to room, pad and pen in hand, making a list of jobs that needed doing. With Lee on tour at the other end of the country (much to his relief, I'm sure), I fortunately had two handymen on call: Martin who is very nifty at putting things together and changing lightbulbs (yes, I still struggle with them) and Duncan who's super-handy with a paintbrush. Until now I'd been happy with the dark rock-and-roll vibe in my flat, but as the nursery was taking on a girly theme the rest of the decor didn't match. I decided every room needed brightening up with at least a lick of paint and while Duncan got busy with his brush, I started to develop an obsession with bleach. As I've mentioned before, I'm obsessed with cleanliness even when I'm not in the grip of pregnancy hormones, but now everything needed going over at least three times.

Poor Lee was next on my hit list as I set about attacking his wardrobe. I was absolutely ruthless and ended up taking bags of his old t-shirts and jeans that I hadn't seen him wearing for months down to the local charity shop. Oh, and don't even get me started on the number of odd socks I found with holes in – and girly pink ones too, I don't wish to know what he was doing with those. To be honest he wasn't too pleased when he returned home on his day off to find his wardrobe half-empty but I think he realised that conflicting with me with my nesting/cleaning head on would not have been conducive to his own health. Luckily after a cuddle and a cup of tea he was soon round to my way of thinking that we'd have lots of fun shopping for replacements.

Cleaning my flat wasn't the only thing I became obsessed with: my teeth had to feel permanently clean too. I'd brush morning, noon and night, and in fact I thought I'd given myself gum disease from brushing too much when my mouth began bleeding heavily. However my dentist reassured me that suffering from sensitive gums is extremely common among pregnant women and advised me to ease off on the manic brushing. Armed with a softer toothbrush and special toothpaste for sensitive gums it cleared up in no time, thank goodness, otherwise photo shoots may have been a problem with my two front teeth missing.

Despite all of nature's little foibles kicking in, every day I was becoming more excited about meeting our little girl and becoming a mum. It's very easy to get caught in a little bubble of joy at times when you're pregnant and forget about the reality that awaits, but when I received a panicked call from my friend Karen to say she was in A&E with her baby daughter Rose I realised I still had some preparing to do for my future life as a mum. Karen had been feeding Rose solid food for the very first time when she began to choke. Karen froze at first before picking Rose up, turning her upside down and patting her firmly on the back until she had coughed the food up. In a panic and wanting to get her checked over, she'd dashed to the hospital with Rose to get the all-clear. Luckily, Rose was fine.

To be honest, these kinds of emergencies and such dangers hadn't even crossed my mind until now so, shaken up by what had happened, Karen and I decided to attend a first-aid course for babies. The tuition was absolutely invaluable and I can't recommend it enough, but I am ashamed to say that I did behave like a naughty schoolgirl whenever I was asked to demonstrate a scenario with a plastic doll (well, you shouldn't ask an actress if you're not expecting things to be hammed up just a bit). I did take a little video camera with me so I could make copies for both Karen and I so we could refer to it at any point but it most definitely won't be appearing on my show reel any time soon.

With just six weeks left until Teapot was due I decided now was a good time to pack my hospital bag, as a lot of my friends' babies had come early and I didn't want to get caught out. I'd been given a list of the necessities I needed to pack by the hospital, which I found really useful. I then set about getting together all the other things I wanted to take with me. I ticked off everything on the list and then kept on going – in fact I think it's fair to say I went slightly overboard, as by the time I'd finished it looked more like I was going on a three-week round-the-world cruise than a trip to the hospital to give birth. PJs, slippers, leggings, flip-flops, tracksuit bottoms, Sudoku, hair straighteners and snacks – every pocket was bulging with things I probably wouldn't need but wanted to take with me just in case. I kept adding things to it, taking everything out and re-packing it to make sure I hadn't forgotten a thing, each time placing it at the bottom of the bed and telling myself I was fully prepared and didn't need anything else.

The evening before the launch of my Very maternity range I was both excited and nervous. It would be the first time the press had seen my collection and even though I loved it, there was no guarantee that it would be positively received. Needless to say my hot flushes, toilet trips and wriggling bump made for a sleepless night, but despite my weariness I arrived at the London Hotel the next morning with a spring in my step. This was a huge day for me; I'd always wanted to design my own range of clothes and, despite the real hard work done by the brilliant creative team at Very, this did still feel like my project – my baby, in fact. The Very team had done a great job of decking out the room and there was tea and cupcakes for guests as they arrived. I was so proud to see two stunning pregnant models wearing my designs to show them off, as up until then I'd only seen them on myself. This now gave me validation that the choices we had made were absolutely perfect and I could totally see my designs being worn by real mums-to-be. As I gave back-to-back interviews with each journalist the feedback on the range was great and the questions about my own pregnancy came rolling out. Are you planning on a natural birth? Would you like to breastfeed? Are you going to have another one after this one? It was so funny, we hadn't even had Teapot yet and everyone wanted to know when the next one was planned.

Now for the Experts...

Exercises to help your baby get in the right position

Any time from Week Thirty-four until the birth, your baby's head will 'engage' and move down into your pelvis. It's often later for those who are carrying a large baby, or one in the posterior position (see below). It may also be later if you have a narrow pelvis or strong stomach muscles. If you are having a second or subsequent baby, it may not engage until labour starts.

If you spend a lot of time sitting down or work in a sedentary job, you are more likely to find that your baby has adopted a posterior position, which means the back of your baby's head and spine is lying against your spine. Unfortunately this can make for a slower and more painful labour with severe back pain. It can also increase the need for an assisted delivery (medical speak for extra intervention such as the use of forceps or a Caesarean).

It's worth, therefore, doing everything you can to get your baby into the 'head-down' anterior position before it engages. To do this you need to keep your pelvis tilted forward as much as possible, which encourages the heaviest part of your baby – the back of its head and spine – to swing round to the front. Babies can change position once they've engaged, but it's obviously easier to turn them before they're in the pelvis. So from about thirty-four weeks, try the following strategies to increase your chances of an anterior baby.

* Sit with your **knees lower than your hips** whenever you can. You can use a cushion to help tilt you forward. Avoid lounging back on your sofa for hours, however attractive a proposition that is!

* When sitting at a desk, use an **upright, firm chair** and try to lean forwards, with your legs slightly apart. You can also use a specialist kneeling chair or large balance ball to sit on.

* Get up and **walk around** every half hour if you are spending a long time sitting down.

* **Kneel** with your palms against a wall and 'walk' your knees backwards so that you are propped leaning forwards with your thighs further back than your hips.

* **Sit back** on your haunches with a pillow under your knees.

* Spend up to ten minutes a day on **all fours** or crawling around, if you feel able to do this. This moves the baby well forward in your pelvis so that the back of the baby's head swings to the front of your abdomen.

Eating to avoid gum disease

During pregnancy you expect to feel bigger and get tired. But you might experience some other changes in your body that are more of a surprise. One of these is something that Denise suffered from, and that's **gingivitis**. This is when your gums become more sensitive and prone to inflammation. One of the symptoms of this is when your gums start bleeding when you brush your teeth. It happens due to hormonal changes in your body – but the good news is that it is reversible. It's important that you do take action, though, as gingivitis can turn into the more serious problem known as **periodontitis**, which can affect the bone in your jaw leading to loose teeth that can end up falling out.

Luckily, if you have an NHS dentist, dental treatment is free during pregnancy so you can go and get expert advice on how to deal with your gums. This will probably involve a session with a hygienist for some thorough cleansing and education regarding tooth brushing techniques, flossing and so on.

As far as prevention is concerned, obviously all gum disease is caused by plaque, a sticky build-up of bacteria that coats both our teeth and gums on a daily basis. So one of the first dietary changes you can make at home is to **cut back on sugary foods** (if you are still eating them), especially between meals. Bacteria in plaque, such as *streptococcus mutans*, stick to our teeth where they need sugars to grow. A coating of sugar from sweets, cakes, biscuits, sweetened teas and coffees, fizzy drinks and squashes provides just that.

Chewing **sugar-free gums** or sucking sweets containing the natural sweetener called xylitol (in Orbit chewing gum for instance) appears to help keep plaque production under control by helping to stop bacteria from sticking to teeth and gums. It also increases saliva flow and makes saliva more alkaline, both of which reduce plaque production. Chewing Orbit after and between meals is certainly worth trying.

Eating products containing **cranberries** may also be helpful. These berries are rich in a type of super-nutrient tannin (known as PACS) that acts as a kind of non-stick coating in various parts of our bodies, helping to stop bacteria from being able to grab on to surfaces like the lining of our urinary tract, and also, it appears, our teeth and gums. Research suggests that using mouthwashes containing these cranberry extracts may help in the treatment of gum disease.

Also check that you are eating **vitamin C-rich** foods each day. It is rare to find people in the UK today with full-blown scurvy (a disease which occurs when we eat very little of this vital nutrient), but in my clinical practice I am sometimes surprised that daily intakes do not hit the daily 40 mg target. Just one medium-sized orange provides double this, while three slices of red pepper in a salad or a kiwi fruit give us 36 mg. Eat 'five a day' of fruit and vegetables and you should easily be covered.

Flavonoids, a group of super-nutrients found in everything from grapefruit, cherries and apples to onions and tea, may also help. Flavonoids were discovered back in the 1930s when they were identified initially as 'vitamin P' because it was found that they helped to keep blood vessels healthy. This role could help to speed up the healing process while their natural antibacterial effects may help to counter gum-attacking bacteria.

Other good flavonoid-rich foods include aubergines, berries, black grapes, parsley, pears, olives, cherry tomatoes, citrus fruits and cabbage.

Eating to avoid varicose veins

One of those consequences of pregnancy that Denise happily avoided was varicose veins. If they run in your family, then you might have a higher chance of getting them at this time in your life. This is because there is extra blood flowing around your body while you are pregnant that puts extra pressure on the veins in your legs – which are already working hard to return blood to your heart.

From a nutritional point of view there are some things you can do which may help, though to date there is no good clinical research to prove this for sure.

The first is to try hard to get on top of **constipation**. Straining to go to the loo can create a build-up of pressure in your entire body, including your circulation. Follow the advice in Chapter Six on how to keep your digestive system healthy.

Another suggestion is to eat plenty of **vitamin C-rich foods** within your 'five a day' of fruits and vegetables. We need vitamin C to help keep the walls of our blood vessels strong and elastic, and this may just help in the battle against varicose veins. Foods rich in vitamin C include nearly all berries, citrus fruits, dark green vegetables, kiwi fruits, papaya and peppers, as well as potatoes and frozen peas.

Spider veins may also be helped by eating foods rich in vitamin C because they are caused by the walls of tiny blood vessels (known as capillaries) rupturing, often under the strain of the extra blood flow. Spider veins are the tiny little red veins that branch out from a central point, often on the face or legs. They are not dangerous and may fade naturally after you've given birth.

Foods rich in dark purple pigments (such as **blueberries** and **aubergines**) may also help by strengthening your blood vessel walls. Other super nutrients that may help to strengthen vein walls can be found in purple sprouting broccoli, red cabbage, red onions and Lollo rosso lettuce.

Further advice to reduce the occurrence of varicose and thread veins includes:

* ❊ **Avoid standing up** for too long.

* ❊ **Walk** as much as possible to get your blood flowing efficiently back up your legs to your heart.

* ❊ Put your **feet up** when sitting (but don't sit for too long or sit with your legs crossed).

* ❊ Wear **support stockings** if your doctor suggests this.

* ❊ If varicose veins don't disappear after delivery, **surgical treatments** are an option.

A word on raspberry leaf tea

Raspberry leaf tea has been given to pregnant women by herbal and traditional practitioners for many centuries. Some believe it stimulates and tones the uterus in preparation for labour, but it is known that taking it before thirty-four weeks can increase the risk of miscarriage. Don't use raspberry leaf tea without first consulting your GP.

Chapter Eleven

Waddle

Month Nine of Pregnancy

What's going on in your body?

Well, it's the home straight now! If your baby hasn't engaged already, it's likely to do so around Week Thirty-six, and you may find yourself adopting that distinctive legs-akimbo late-pregnancy waddle. You may also need to pee constantly as your uterus drops and presses against your bladder, and you may suffer from round ligament pain at the front of your bump when you walk. Your baby will be around 47 cm long at the start of this month and will weigh about 2.6 kg, rising to an average of 51 cm and 3.4 kg at full term, so even in those last four weeks he will be putting on weight at a rate of knots. At Week Thirty-eight your baby's lanugo (fine hair) will start dropping off his body, though some babies still have a smattering of this at birth. As for you, you may be in full-on 'nesting' mode in the run-up to birth, or just simply sick of the whole thing and desperate for it to be over.

Your baby is considered 'full-term' from Week Thirty-eight. Forty weeks is the average length of pregnancy (thirty-seven for twins), but of course some go on a week or two longer. Every pregnancy is different and there is no obvious predictor for when you will go into labour.

So all you have to do now is wait…

My Diary

ust four weeks left until my due date and I felt as though my baby could arrive at any time. Surely she was getting short of space in there? Every time she moved my belly looked like a scene from *Alien* with a hand or foot appearing pressed against my skin like it could burst through at any minute. Loads of my friends have had early babies, in particular my sister-in-law who gave birth to my beautiful niece Freja six weeks early, so any fears I had about an early arrival were starting to dissipate in favour of genuine excitement that it wouldn't be long before we got to meet our little girl. I knew now that even if she arrived tomorrow she'd be healthy and gorgeous, and with that change of mindset comes an amazing feeling of relief and happiness.

I was finding hundreds of chores to do around the house to keep me busy and on the move. If Lee sat still long enough I'd have vacuumed the curls out of his hair – I just had to do anything so I wasn't sitting around waiting for a twinge or my waters to break. I'd heard the last month of pregnancy described as a halfway house and now I was starting to understand why: you're too pregnant to work as hard as you're used to but you still need to find reasons to keep busy. In an attempt to remain my usual super-organised self I filled the cupboards in the flat with all the things I knew I'd need once I left hospital. I had enough washing powder, teabags, choccie biscuits and loo rolls to see me through the next year let alone a few weeks. I also cooked a couple of meals and popped them in the freezer to make sure I had something nutritious to eat if I couldn't be bothered to cook when I got home.

I'd learned from Karen's experiences that I may not want to see a whole queue of people as soon as Teapot arrived, but I didn't want to risk it being another six months before I did see everyone. So I figured the best thing to do at this point would be to get everyone together for one big gathering, a girly get-together of massive proportions – yes, a baby shower. Just the name 'baby shower' gives away that it's an American concept but despite being a bit of a traditionalist at heart I have no shame in saying it's a fantastic idea for any expectant mum and in my opinion we don't celebrate enough over here in Blighty. I went to lots of showers when I was living in Los Angeles and they were always great fun and the perfect opportunity for the mum-to-be to be spoilt for the day. There's usually a strict 'no men allowed' rule but I broke it (only slightly) by inviting two of my gay friends along to mine.

I wanted it to be as intimate as possible yet despite my best attempts to keep the numbers down I was still left with forty guests I really wanted to see, so we took over the Cibo Café at Mamas and Papas in central London. It was a really special afternoon with little girls running everywhere, all wearing beautiful fairy wings (one of the conditions of entry for the kids), and while the adults tucked in to a spread of food and champagne the little ones kept themselves busy by decorating fairy cakes and colouring.

Like most girlie gatherings, once the champagne had been flowing for a while it was time to play a few games, with 'Guess the Flavour of the Baby Food' going down well. Needless to say, my friends who are already mums had a huge advantage and won hands-down. Teapot was spoilt rotten with loads of wonderful presents, and there were so many lovely outfits for her that there was now a serious risk of me getting wardrobe envy.

I can guarantee that if you have a baby shower and your friends spoil you with lots of gifts for you and your baby, one of the first things your man will say is, 'What about me?' It's a given that they're going to feel a bit left out, so my advice would be to plan something romantic for just the two of you before the baby arrives. Lee and I had another excuse to plan something special because later that week we celebrated our first wedding anniversary. Lee was so excited and wanted to celebrate by doing something really amazing, but seeing as I felt like I was the size of a house and was rapidly becoming too tired to handle late nights I wasn't so keen to do anything too extravagant or to go too far. In the end we opted for low-key and local at my favourite Italian restaurant around the corner from the flat. Over our dinner of pasta, pasta and more pasta we spent the whole time reminiscing on how fast the year had flown by and how grateful we both were to have a baby on the way. It's amazing just how quickly everything had happened – marriage and a baby all within a single year – though I wouldn't have wanted it any other way.

Needless to say my hubby was ever the gentleman throughout the evening and kept telling me how beautiful I looked, but even his sincerity couldn't convince me as I still felt huge and unattractive. It's not just the increase in weight that makes you look and feel larger but also the swelling – I was definitely not prepared for my hands and feet taking on a life of their own. By this point too I was still wearing both my wedding and engagement rings as I hadn't realised just how fast my hands would blow up. They were literally fine one day and then the next I had pork sausage fingers and my rings weren't coming off without ring cutters. I cannot advise you strongly enough to remove any jewellery as soon as you notice any swelling in your hands.

I went for my last trip to our house in Kent and spent most of the time laughing at myself as I thoroughly cleaned everything to make sure it was tidy for Teapot's first visit. Of course she wouldn't know any different if there was washing up in the sink or the pictures weren't straight, but it mattered to me. I also spent lots of time in the garden planting sunflowers and daisies in the hope that they would grow with her and she would enjoy looking at them when she was a few months old. It was weird knowing that the next time I would be there would be with our little girl.

So with the bags all packed and ready, the houses tidied and the kitchen cupboards stocked up, it was now time for some last-minute preening. My belly now being the size of a beach ball meant I could see very little of my lower body but I wasn't going to use this as an excuse to resemble a hippy, so I booked in for a bikini wax to make sure I looked presentable down below for the big day. It seems so ludicrous even mentioning this now but it felt important at the time. Now what was it to be? A Brazilian (just a strip of hair), Hollywood (all off) or an Essex (backcombed with highlights)? Whatever she gave me it felt much better, even though I was unable to admire her handiwork myself.

Six days before my due date I began to feel a dull ache close to my pubic bone. I dismissed it at first as my body preparing itself for the nearing birth, but the following day the pains had got worse and I was feeling very uncomfortable, so I called my obstetrician Pat to tell him. He asked me to pop in to see him there and then. Could this be it? Could we really be getting ready to meet Teapot within the next day or so? Pat checked me over and told me he wasn't happy with the way the baby was sitting and he'd feel happier if I were to have a Caesarean section – and as I was suffering from the pain and swelling he would be happy to perform the operation the following day. To say that this came as a shock would be an understatement. After nine months of mentally preparing for the birth this was a real curveball and to be honest I wasn't sure what to do. I called Lee immediately to explain what had happened and after talking it over we decided we should take the doctor's expert advice and do what was best for the baby.

Rebecca the midwife and my friends who have already been through it had warned me not to pin my hopes on everything going to plan when it came to the birth, because nine times out of ten there will be a spanner in the works. I must admit to feeling a little bit disappointed that I wasn't going to give birth naturally, especially as I'd been religiously practising my deep breathing, but my main concern was that Teapot arrived safe and sound. I'd also been told that, no matter what happens, as soon as your baby arrives healthy and you hear them crying for the first time, you soon forget everything you've been through.

There had been a pack of photographers waiting across the street from my flat for the past few days, poised ready to catch a snap of me scrambling to the car mid-contraction. As sorry as I feel for them having to camp out day and night for days on end, I had to throw them off the scent, so I went off to my mate Lucy's house to stay for the evening. Hanging out with one of my dearest friends was actually a lovely thing to do and we spent the evening chatting, raking over old times when we were footloose and fancy-free and taking some last-minute pictures of my enormous bump.

I woke up the next morning ready for action. This was it: D-Day! Everything we had been working towards in the past nine or ten months was here – the moment I had been cleaning for, decorating for, in fact this was the day I had been working for my whole life. I was finally going to become a mum. As Lucy drove me to the hospital we had a good laugh when she turned on the radio and out blasted Diana Ross singing, 'I'm coming out, I want the world to know...' I couldn't have picked a better song for the journey. I reached the hospital to find Lee waiting for me with a huge smile on his face, holding the day's newspapers that I'd asked him to buy so we could save them for when Teapot was older.

When I got to my room I carefully unpacked all of the little baby things I'd brought with me and stashed away my snacks for later. I felt a complete fool putting on the hospital gown with the ties at the back, fearing my bottom could poke out at any moment. All the time I was cracking jokes and felt really calm, which took me by surprise – I would have thought that by now I'd be breathing into a paper bag or having a go at the gas and air to calm my nerves. It was actually Lee who had the jitters, probably because he'd never spent time in hospital for anything so the whole situation was a little bit alien for him.

I had the high-dose epidural administered, which took a few minutes to kick in. That was the most bizarre sensation, gradually losing the feeling in my lower half before it went totally numb. Lee popped on the CD we'd put together as our 'birth-day' playlist. After a great deal of deliberation we went for a Burt Bacharach compilation and had joked that she'd most likely make an appearance to 'Raindrops Keep Fallin' on My Head'. Lo and behold, that's exactly what happened. I couldn't quite believe she'd arrived. Thanks to the high-definition scans I'd had, she looked exactly how I'd imagined her to, and I instantly felt like I recognised her.

Absolutely beaming with pride, looking both professional and handsome in his scrubs, Lee cut the umbilical cord. I was laughing my head off because he looked like a hunky doctor in a hospital drama. Give me Lee over George Clooney any day.

Our beautiful little girl had finally arrived, slightly earlier than planned, but safe and sound. With no word of a lie, as soon as she was presented to me swaddled in a blanket, the song 'Magic Moments' cued up on the CD and brought a smile to everyone's faces in the operating theatre. She looked perfect and was so warm and tiny. I could feel contentment radiating from her and I fell instantly in love. Lee and I just stared at her as she gave us a little pout (which I promptly named the Portland Pout). There was no doubt she looked just like the name we'd had for her all along – Betsy Mead.

The first of May 2010, the day Betsy arrived, was the best day of my life. My friends had tried to describe the feeling to me in the past but I hadn't quite got it. I have experienced so many massive highs throughout my career so I was sure it would be a similar feeling to what I'd experienced before, but nothing even comes close to how you feel the day you hold your own newborn baby.

Now for the Experts...

If, unlike Denise, you have reached full term and there are no complications, you may be looking for ways to bring on labour naturally. We've all heard the ones about hot curries and sex – but how about cuddling a newborn baby or even a nice bit of nipple-tweaking?

There are varying degrees of medical truth behind these theories but as none of them can do any harm once you're full term you might as well go for it! However, there is one thing you can easily do to encourage your baby to descend and to trigger labour, and that is exercise. Try the following to help speed things along:

Walking

This keeps you upright and helps your baby's head to engage. As well as being good for you, walking exerts downward pressure on your cervix, which can help dilation and increases the release of oxytocin, the hormone responsible for kick-starting contraction. (Oxytocin can also be released when you cuddle a newborn, have an orgasm or have your nipples tweaked, hence the theories mentioned above!)

Climbing stairs

This is another great way to get your baby to engage better, to dilate your cervix and to increase the oxytocin levels in your cervical area. In addition, the act of lifting your legs to climb actually opens up your pelvis and helps your baby to get in a good position for labour. In fact, midwives sometimes ask women to walk up and down stairs to help speed up labour if things aren't progressing well. Just don't go crazy and exhaust yourself.

Swimming

As outlined on pages 116–18, swimming is a great method of exercising in pregnancy. It can also help to relieve the problem of swelling in your hands and feet if, like Denise, you are suffering from this.

Squatting

This helps to open the pelvis and encourages your baby to descend in the correct position for birth. Squatting can also speed up labour by encouraging the baby down the birth canal more quickly.

Swinging

Yes it's true, a nice gentle swing in the park can result in a small G-force that encourages your baby to descend! But whatever you do, make sure the swing is safe and stable before you get on it – after all, you are likely to be weighing considerably more than the small child it was designed for!

Eating and drinking during labour

Different people have different opinions about whether it's safe to eat once your labour is established; some hospitals don't allow it, so check with your midwife what the policy is. In general, doctors worry about it as a full stomach may cause complications if you end up needing an epidural, pethidine or a Caesarean, whereas midwives often worry if women are *not* allowed to eat in labour, as after all you'll be using up a lot of energy and it can go on a long time. In fact, you can become dizzy and faint or dehydrated if you don't eat anything at all.

As ever, a sensible midway policy is normally the best solution – in other words, eat if you are hungry in early labour, but stick to light, easily digestible food such as soup, scrambled egg, toast or cereals. Once your labour is established, listen to your body and ask the advice of your medical team if you are not sure: you are unlikely to be hungry when in strong labour in any case.

The main thing is to make sure you keep well hydrated throughout labour, as it can slow down if you become dehydrated. Drink regularly or suck on ice cubes if drinking is uncomfortable. Pack some sports drinks or glucose tablets in your hospital bag and take those if you need an extra burst of energy. You can also drink fruit juice or squashes to raise your blood sugar levels if you are feeling faint. However, the most important thing is to listen to the advice of your midwife and medical team, because every birth is different.

Chapter Twelve

Swaddle
Betsy's First Month

What's going on in your body?

You did it! And however you did it – whether it was a natural home-birth lit with scented candles or a full-on emergency Caesarean complete with flashing blue lights, you deserve a tremendous pat on the back. Bringing a new life into the world is an extraordinary achievement.

The days immediately after the birth will be a blur of excitement: getting to know your beautiful new baby (surely the most gorgeous ever created?), fending off endless visitors, getting to grips with breastfeeding – or not as the case may be, dealing with the most extraordinarily revolting nappies (newborn poo – known as meconium – is greenish-black and tar-like), and wondering whether your life will ever be normal again (the short answer: no, not for a long while). You may find yourself virtually hallucinating through lack of sleep, and experiencing wild hormonal changes that make your mood swing from elation to despair in the space of minutes. You may also be in pain after the birth: at best you are likely to be bruised; at worst you may have had stitches or a Caesarean. You will also have a heavy period-like bleed for a few weeks after the birth: this is normal and should reduce gradually after the first week, though tell your midwife if the bleeding suddenly becomes heavy or clotted.

Your baby may also not look quite how you had envisaged – the umbilical stump can seem rather odd, his head might be slightly squashed from birth, his genitals might seem huge thanks to the effect of your hormones on his body, he may have 'stork marks' (red marks on his face or neck), or vernix or lanugo covering the skin. All these things should settle down after a few weeks. And in any case, didn't we already establish your newborn is the most beautiful baby ever?

So, congratulations. Your new life starts here…

My Diary

Once the medical team had completed all of the relevant health checks I was wheeled back up to my room, with Lee riding shotgun. We were left alone in the privacy of our little sanctuary and it was such a special time, the first moments we were ever going to spend together as a new family. Not quite believing she was finally here, we sat in awe, staring at our baby daughter. She looked so perfect, and although she weighed a healthy 7 lb 10 oz she seemed so tiny and fragile. Her gorgeous blue eyes were melting me already and her brown hair already had a slight curl to it, definitely taking after her dad in that department. I felt so content sitting with my lovely husband cooing over baby Betsy and she seemed just as content to be with us.

I can't say anything negative about the birth at all, it was a magical experience – however I was not expecting my nipples to start feeling like someone had just stubbed cigarettes out on them. So when the midwife turned up to help me breastfeed I was a little wary to say the least. Although by this time the burning sensation had subsided, leaving an uncomfortable sting, it seems my pre-birth naïvety of thinking that breastfeeding would be easy was a little off-track. No one had mentioned beforehand the things we women are faced with when trying this for the first time. Difficulty getting the baby to latch on; not producing enough milk; painful nipples – all these things can happen to anyone. In fact my midwife told me that the best breastfeeding mums are the ones that aren't bothered whether or not they succeed at first because they put less pressure on themselves and are therefore more relaxed as a result. Thanks to the extreme patience and support of my midwife I managed to get the hang of it and Betsy began to feed nicely, fortunately putting an end to the high-pitched screaming that the little madam had discovered was a very effective way of letting us know she was hungry. Still, at least we knew she had a good set of lungs on her.

Once Betsy was content and sleeping I took the opportunity to call my family to let them know she'd arrived and we were doing great. Of course my parents were eager to meet Betsy as soon as possible but we agreed that the following day would be best, to give me a chance to get some much-needed rest. Next I set about texting everyone in my mobile's address book to share the good news – and I do mean everyone. I must have still been slightly under the influence of the drugs I'd been given before the operation because I sent messages to people I hadn't been in touch with for years. So I'd like to take this opportunity to apologise to anyone who received a random 'She's arrived!' message, including Susan at Hamptons Estate Agents who I know definitely received one from me (oh, and Susan, if you are reading this, I'm still very happy with the flat you sold me six years ago, thank you).

Four hours after my operation and on the advice of my doctor I was up on my feet and walking around. I was keen to speed up my recovery in any way I could, without overdoing it of course, and was really surprised at how mobile I was, bearing in mind I'd been on the operating table just that morning.

So as our big day came to a close the three of us settled down in our room to watch some Saturday night telly while tucking into a huge margherita pizza (well, Betsy didn't indulge in the pizza of course – I had her share – but she did seem to enjoy *Britain's Got Talent*). Throughout the evening, as I held our new daughter, my emotions would wash over me, leaving me feeling overwhelmed. I was experiencing a love that I had never felt before, different from that which I felt for Lee or my family.

Throughout the night Betsy did her fair share of exercising her lungs – I guess she was just making sure they worked properly and making up for all the time she couldn't shout at me from in the womb. I did manage to drift off eventually, and waking up in the morning was like Christmas day as I peered over to see her little face. It's hard to explain the feelings I experienced, I just wish that exact emotion could be captured and bottled to share it around.

This was to be our first dressing-up session – not quite old enough for angel wings and princess dresses yet but I did find her cutest babygrow for her to meet her grandparents in and she looked gorgeous. As the family visited she was passed around and cuddled to within an inch of her life. I felt very emotional watching everyone holding her and cooing over her, and just felt blessed that she was going to have so much love in her life as she grew up.

By day three in the hospital all of our family had done the rounds and gone home in love with Betsy, and unfortunately Lee had to leave us to go back to work. I'd been getting on fine squeezing my nipple and popping the colostrum into Betsy's mouth but things soon changed. I was thankful I had opted to stay in hospital because on day three my boobs were enormous and really painful. One of the nurses explained to me that it meant my milk had come in. That's all well and good but I had a couple of prize-winning melons on my chest: what was I supposed to do with them? On her instruction I took a hot bath and placed a warm wet flannel across my chest and squeezed milk from both of my boobs into the bath which definitely helped relieve the pressure a bit but was no miracle cure.

No matter how much I tried Betsy just wouldn't latch onto my nipple and would cry uncontrollably. She was hungry and I was getting frustrated, wondering what I was doing wrong. Stressed and upset, I called my mum who explained that she breastfed my sister who was first born with no problem whatsoever. My brother was next to arrive and was such a greedy baby that she couldn't keep up with the demand and ended up moving to formula. By the time I came along my mum had two toddlers running around and just didn't have time to sit down and breastfeed, so I was bottle fed from the off and didn't turn out too bad. Despite all the books I'd read and the despite the midwife offering her advice it was only my mum's words that reassured me that not everyone is able to breastfeed for a variety of reasons. As the saying goes, mum really does know best.

Thankfully, on the advice of my mummy friends I had kept the day pretty free, as they had explained that it would be likely that I was to come down off my massive high around that time. They were so right and a wave of emotion and exhaustion washed over me at the same time. Out of nowhere I started crying uncontrollably, not because I was feeling sad but a mixture of tiredness and joy. Throughout the day the nurse kept popping in to make sure I was OK and explained that it was completely natural to feel emotional at this point. I told her that I felt silly because I wasn't feeling miserable but was unable to control my tears, and she assured me that each woman goes through a different experience. In fact there was a woman the same age as me a few doors down who gave birth on the same day I did but I'd heard she wasn't coping very well with it all. Her emotions had kicked in along with feelings of nervousness and an inability to cope – she felt like she was unable to look after the baby and wasn't prepared for motherhood. It's a very common feeling in the early days after you've given birth, apparently. I never got to meet her but I hope that her worries eventually calmed down and she had as much joy from her new baby as I was now getting from little Betsy. One thing I learned from that day was the importance of sharing your feelings with the people around you while on this emotional rollercoaster, especially the medical staff who can put your mind at rest by assuring you you're not going mad.

Over the next few days I stayed in hospital where the nurses helped me with Betsy and made sure I knew how to change, bath and care for her properly, so by the time I was due to leave I was confident in looking after her myself. However when the time came for me to step outside the little bubble I'd been in, I still felt like I was heading into the unknown.

No matter how much planning and preparation you make before you go into hospital you can't account for everything when you return home. I pulled up outside my front door to discover my upstairs neighbours had given permission for maintenance work to be undertaken on the outside of our house, so I was greeted by scaffolding covering the whole building, allowing very little light into my ground-floor flat, and workmen sitting having a cuppa and a fag in my garden. Let's just say those deep breathing exercises I had practised for labour came in extremely useful in calming myself down before I hit the roof.

The following day my midwife unexpectedly turned up on the doorstep to make sure I was coping with Betsy and to weigh her. Seeing her at my home just gave me another little boost of confidence because despite all the guidance and magazines I'd read over the past nine months I always seemed to have questions about whether I was doing everything properly. Thankfully I'd managed to take a shower and brush my hair, which was a challenge in itself, so I didn't look like I'd been dragged through a hedge backwards (aka my usual morning look). During the early days of my pregnancy I had promised myself that I would continue to make an effort to look presentable once I became a mum as my friends had warned me how easy it is to stay in a dressing gown all day and tuck into biscuits and cakes while watching daytime TV. I wanted to keep my spirits up by feeling good about myself, eating healthily and making sure I didn't pile on any extra pounds now when I still had quite a few still to lose. It's funny because I had half-expected my body to return to normal pretty quickly and had been looking forward to wearing my regular clothes again, but my body was taking its time – so there was no throwing away the boulder-holder bras and elasticated waistbands just yet. Meanwhile the latest addition to my wardrobe – a pair of control pants – was doing a great job of hiding my jelly belly.

Over the next few days my friends started to visit, kindly bringing little treats like coffee and cake (well, the odd indulgence doesn't hurt). We had so many visitors all bearing gifts and flowers that, at one point, we placed Betsy centre-stage in the middle of the room in her Moses basket and joked that she was as popular as baby Jesus.

When my friend Sam visited, proudly sporting her six-month pregnancy bump, it was my turn to try to explain the feelings you experience as a new mum meeting your baby for the first time. The love that's different from anything you have felt before and the feeling of contentment. I also warned her about a few of the things I wasn't expecting, such as the big long greeny-black poo that comes out soon after baby puts in an appearance, which took me by surprise (it's called meconium and is made up of materials the baby has taken in while inside the uterus), and of course the fiery nipples.

With Betsy centre of attention and me not doing too badly for treats when we had visitors, I wanted to make sure Lee didn't feel neglected. His opening night in the West End show *Wicked* was the perfect opportunity to let him know how special he was to us. With him busy juggling fatherhood with work I thought he could do with a spot of pampering, so I bought him a voucher for a massage. On the card I wrote, 'To Daddy, good luck in your new show, lots of love Betsy.' Needless to say it was greeted with smiles and went down a treat.

Each day got easier as I became accustomed to working my life around Betsy's schedule. When Betsy was sleeping I'd catch up on chores and emails and even sneak in the odd snooze too. I was getting the hang of it until we hit week three when everything seemed to change. Betsy began to cry uncontrollably every time I tried to put her down – it was exhausting. I've heard so many conflicting opinions about leaving babies to cry. Is it best to let them settle themselves sometimes or are they trying to tell you they need something? I didn't really know what to do at this point. Unless I was holding her in my arms she just wasn't happy, and before long my back was killing me, my arms were aching and I had dark circles under my eyes. It was then that I realised it wasn't going to be all plain sailing and during that week I had a couple of mummy meltdowns where I sat on the bed – which was still unmade because I couldn't put Betsy down – and just cried. I was learning a very important lesson that I'm sure most new mums realise eventually, which was to accept help whenever it was offered. My mum was great and would pop around whenever she could to allow me a bit of freedom to have a soak in the bath or even just to escape to the local shop for a pint of milk. I've never appreciated that five-minute walk so much.

I've learnt, and am still learning, that motherhood isn't always easy. It's a bumpy, twisty, turning road that can take its toll from time to time. Yet all the sleepless nights and ear-shattering cries from Betsy are totally outweighed by a single smile or by watching her eyelids softly close as she gets milk-drunk.

The last bit of sage advice from my friends who have helped me so much on my journey so far: they grow up quickly – so enjoy the time.

I intend to, every minute of it.

Now for the Experts...

How to get your body back in shape after the birth

OK, so you've just given birth, so you don't want to hear about exercising just yet – it's hard enough just to get up and get dressed. But there will come a time when a vague daydream of getting your old body back will flicker across your mind – and then is the time to take action. Exercise is great for boosting your confidence and self-esteem, and helping you to combat the baby blues and even postnatal depression. So by taking some small steps at first, you will soon find yourself on your way back to looking fabulous and feeling great again (hmm, let's just settle for 'normal' at first).

You can do pelvic floor exercises within a day or so of having your baby, but wait around six weeks before you do any 'proper' exercise, assuming you've had an uncomplicated pregnancy and birth – possibly longer if you had a Caesarean like Denise. Speak to your doctor or midwife if you're not sure whether you're ready yet. Whenever you start, go easy on yourself, and stop if you feel any pain or discomfort, or if your post-birth bleeding becomes heavier or starts up again after having previously stopped (if you have any fresh red blood, see your doctor).

Remember that if you're breastfeeding you'll need to be extra-careful about overdoing it as otherwise it may affect your milk supply.

Starting exercising after you've given birth

Little and often

You're unlikely to have time to exercise continuously for an hour at a time once your baby has arrived, but remember that every little helps. Even just a **ten-minute session** every morning and afternoon will make a difference. You can even do your pelvic floor exercises when you breastfeed!

Make your home a gym

Your living room will probably resemble a cross between the baby section of a department store and a florist by now, but try to **clear a space** to put a mat down for you to do some floor exercises. Your baby can sit alongside you while you work out, in a carrycot or bouncy chair, or on his own playmat.

Do the baby workout

If, like Denise, you have a baby that doesn't like to be put down, why not **incorporate him** into your routine? Most babies love being danced around the room to music, and you can even use him as a free weight! Try lying on your back on the floor, knees bent, with your baby resting on your chest. Then carefully lift him up and down to work your arms. Alternatively hold your baby facing outwards, close to your chest, as you lean back against a wall. From this position you can do squats to tone your thighs and bottom.

Get outside

It's very easy to cocoon yourself at home after you've given birth, but it's important for both you and the baby that you get regular **fresh air**. It might be too early at the moment for you to join one of those 'prambusting' jogging sessions in the local park, but you can still make an effort to walk briskly when you next take the buggy to the local shops. If you want to increase your strength, you could even wear little ankle weights – or of course you could put your baby in a sling or back carrier to build up your back muscles!

Meet other mums

It's really worth getting yourself on the local 'mummy grapevine' as most areas will have a **postnatal fitness class** in which you can bring your baby along. Sometimes these will be held in local council-run fitness centres, sometimes they're just private classes in church halls, so ask around. If all else fails, why not suggest putting on a workout DVD or going for a brisk walk round the park next time you meet up with one of your new mummy friends? Remember that everyone will be struggling with the same body issues as you so don't be embarrassed to bring it up.

Tummy-busting moves

The first question that any new mum asks about her body is, 'Why is my tummy still so big?' Don't worry, it may feel huge and doughy after you've just given birth, but over time it will gradually shrink back to normal. However, there are still things you can do to help it tone up more quickly and to get rid of the squidgy bits.

The main thing is to focus on your transverse abdominals – the deepest muscles that lie horizontally and act like a girdle round your middle. Having tight transverse abs will help get your rectus abdominus muscles back into place (they often split during pregnancy to accommodate your growing baby), and help you achieve a flatter stomach, better posture and fewer backaches.

Most traditional stomach crunches target your vertical abs, which don't help you to get a flatter tummy. So there's no point in doing endless sit-ups as your transverse muscles will barely feel the effects. Instead concentrate on doing exercises that make you pull your stomach in, such as lunges (in which you keep your back straight by tightening your transverse abdominals). Pilates classes are very good at focusing on this area, but if you can't get to one, here are some suggestions for specific transverse-targeted exercises you can do at home:

Scissor kicks

1 Lie on the floor on your back, with your hands underneath your buttocks to keep your spine flat.
2 Raise one leg about 30 cm off the floor and slowly lower it back down, raising the other as you do so. Aim for three sets of ten repetitions.

Pelvic tilts

1 Still lying on the floor, bend your knees while keeping your feet on the ground.
2 Slowly lift up your pelvis and hold it there briefly, sucking your navel into your spine, before lowering it slowly back down. Keep your upper body on the floor as you do this. Do three sets of fifteen reps.

The no-crunch crunch

1 Lie on the floor as in the previous exercise. Place your hands just below and to the sides of your belly button, on your lower abdomen.

2 Gently draw your lower abs down towards the floor (envisage a piece of string pulling your navel downwards), but do not move your pelvis, raise your chest or hold your breath. You should feel the muscles under your fingers becoming taut, but be careful not to pull in too far because you'll end up working your oblique abs (side muscles) rather than your transverse abs instead. This is an 'easy' exercise but don't worry, it's still doing you good!

3 Hold the position for ten to fifteen seconds, breathing normally the whole time, and aim for ten reps.

Box press-up

1 Turn over so you're on all fours with your hands shoulder-width apart, elbows slightly bent. Keep your knees together under your hips (you can make this exercise more difficult by placing your knees slightly behind you).

2 Curl your toes underneath you onto the floor so your heels point up. Tighten your transverse abs by drawing your navel in to your spine, then slowly raise your knees off the ground so your weight goes into your hands and feet. Your upper body should not move.

3 Hold for one breath then slowly lower down, and aim for three sets of ten.

Eating for breastfeeding

When breastfeeding it makes complete sense to go on eating a healthy and balanced diet. While pregnant you 'feed' your baby with the nutrients transported via your placenta, whereas with breastfeeding you are swapping to feeding him via your milk. Either way, the health of your body and the things you eat and drink can directly affect the health of your growing baby.

This table sets out how many more calories a new mum should eat to support the production of milk while breastfeeding. However, remember that these figures are designed to cover the needs of all breastfeeding women and so are not tailor-made to your needs. It is best, therefore, to use this table as a rough guide, with your own individual appetite and thirst informing your actual needs. Probably, a little bit like during pregnancy, metabolic changes take place in our bodies so that we are still really efficient with calories, which may well reduce the true calorie cost of producing sufficient milk to keep a baby growing well.

Extra calories needed during breastfeeding

Month 1	An extra 450 daily
Month 2	An extra 530 daily
Month 3	An extra 570 daily
Months 4-6	An extra 480 daily if you introduce weaning from four months
Months 4-6	An extra 570 daily if you exclusively breastfeed
Over 6 months	An extra 240 daily if you follow usual weaning procedures
Over 6 months	An extra 550 daily if you continue to provide breast milk as the main source of nourishment.

Extra minerals

To produce good quality breast milk you need plenty of **calcium** in your diet. You can meet the extra 550 mg that you need a day (this is in addition to the usual 700 mg women need daily), by having a pint of skimmed milk or half a pint of skimmed milk and a yoghurt. Other good foods for calcium include sesame seeds, steamed tofu, dried figs, sardines canned in oil, almonds and dark green vegetables.

Along with extra calcium, your body also needs more of another bone-building mineral called **phosphorus**, plus more **magnesium**, **zinc**, **copper** and **selenium**. If you are eating more healthy foods within a balanced diet to meet the extra calorie needs of breastfeeding, you should already be covering these additional requirements.

Extra vitamins

Not surprisingly, during breastfeeding you will also need extra vitamins: in fact you need more of all them, with the exception of vitamin B6. Again, most will be covered by the extra food that you will be eating anyway. However, the government recommends that you take a 10-microgram supplement of **vitamin D** daily, as you might not get enough through your diet alone.

What NOT to eat

When it comes to breastfeeding you need to generally stick with the same rules regarding **fish** as when you were pregnant. However, there are some small changes: for example you can go up to two portions per week of oily fish (e.g. salmon, sardines, pilchards, mackerel, fresh tuna and trout). With reference to swordfish, marlin and shark, you can now have up to one portion per week, although personally – due to the high levels of mercury in these fish – I'd recommend avoiding them altogether for the time being, especially if you are thinking of having another baby at a later date.

Peanuts are fine to eat as long as you don't have an allergy to them yourself. With other foods the best advice is to avoid eating any that you think may be affecting your baby – strong flavours get passed into the breast milk so you may find there are times when your baby seems 'off' his feed after you've eaten something very spicy, for example. That said, one of the benefits of breastfeeding is that the baby is exposed to a wider variety of tastes than if he is bottle-fed, which may help when you come to wean. Certainly you should check with your health visitor before you start permanently excluding foods, especially ones that form a mainstay of your diet such as wheat-based items.

As ever, try to eat regularly and healthily but keep meals simple. Snack on nutritious things like fruit, yoghurts and nuts (if you can eat them) and make sure that you keep your fluid intakes up throughout the day.

Continue to keep **caffeine** in drinks to a minimum while breastfeeding because studies show that caffeine is rapidly transferred into breast milk – and logically, it can't be good for your baby to be getting caffeine highs at such a young age! The same advice of course goes for **alcohol.**

Denise's Top Tips

After the birth, make sure you have:
* Plenty of sanitary towels
* Big (Bridget Jones) knickers
* Loose lounge trousers

Out and about, make sure you carry:
* Muslins and bibs
* Nappies and wipes
* A spare outfit in case of accidents

Things to remember:
* Take lots of pics
* Keep a diary (great to look back on)
* Most importantly – register the birth!

Don't neglect YOU:
* Make time for a soak in a bubble bath
* Have an evening out (or in with your girlfriends)
* Listen to music that makes you happy
* Don't forget – you're amazing... you're a mum!

Index

Acknowledgements

A huge thank you to everyone involved in making this book possible, especially…

Sam Mann, who wrote this book with me – I can't thank you enough for your time and dedication. The past few months have shown me that not only are you a great writer, but also a true friend who never lets me down. I'm so pleased we are now mums and look forward to all the wonderful times we will spend together with our new families. It's great that Betsy and your baby daughter April will grow up together as best friends.

Nicki Waterman and Amanda Ursell, your advice and support throughout my pregnancy was invaluable. I'm so pleased we have the opportunity to share your expertise with as many mums as possible.

Everyone at Headline Publishing, especially Emma Tait and Carly Cook.

My agents Gordon Wise at Curtis Brown and Claire Dundas at ARG.

Simon Jones and the team at Hackford Jones.

My obstetrician Pat O'Brian, Dr Anthony Silverstone and all the lovely midwives at The Portland Hospital who took care of me.

My husband Lee, for putting up with my ever-changing moods throughout my pregnancy and of course his part in making our daughter.

My beautiful daughter Betsy, for making my life complete and of course without whom this book would not have been possible.

All images courtesy of Denise Van Outen except those listed below.
Getty Images: page 2 (top left, top right); page 3 (top right); page 4 (top left, top right)
Tim Griffiths: page 6 (bottom left)
Louis Dundas Centre for Children's Palliative Care at Great Ormond Street Hospital: page 8 (top)